WAKE UP SLEEPY HEAD!

Diagnosing, Understanding, and
Navigating Narcolepsy

Debra J. Stultz M.D.

First published by Ultimate World Publishing 2023
Copyright © 2023 Debra Stultz

ISBN

Paperback: 978-1-923123-03-8
Ebook: 978-1-923123-04-5

Cover design: Ultimate World Publishing
Layout and typesetting: Ultimate World Publishing
Editor: Marnae Kelley
Cover Image Copyright: fizkes-Shutterstock.com
Back Cover Image: Mark Webb Photograpy

Ultimate World Publishing
Diamond Creek,
Victoria Australia 3089
www.writeabook.com.au

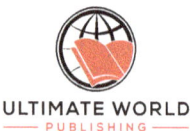

"Those who have compared our life to a dream were right . . .

we were sleeping wake and waking sleep."

Michel de Montaigne

Testimonials

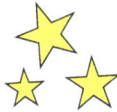

I have had the pleasure of working, researching, studying, and teaching with Dr. Debbie Stultz for many years. She has now translated her years of experience in sleep medicine and psychiatry into a patient-oriented work, which will be invaluable to narcolepsy patients navigating their disorder and treatment course.

Richard K. Bogan, MD, FCCP, FAASM,
Bogan Sleep Consultants, LLC

Dr. Debbie Stultz is one of the most empathetic patient advocates for Narcolepsy I have ever had the privilege of meeting. I have worked with her for the past fifteen years in the field of sleep and Narcolepsy. She is one of the most dedicated and knowledgeable physicians in the field and spends countless hours every week with patients and their families. She understands how debilitating this disease can be on patients' lives and strives daily to make their lives better and more enjoyable.

Jimmy Cunningham, Senior Specialty Consultant,
Jazz Pharmaceuticals

Dr. Stultz's book is an excellent resource for people living with Narcolepsy and their support network. From diagnosis to treatment, you'll get practical insights about every step in the journey. A must-read for anyone affected by Narcolepsy!

Matthew Day, Executive Director of Marketing,
Harmony Biosciences, LLC

Beside the words 'dedicated' and 'compassionate' in the dictionary, there should be a picture of Dr. Stultz. While working with her for six years, I frequently noticed she was the first to arrive and last to leave, working diligently on ways to best help patients near and far. You would want to consult Dr. Stultz for information regarding the sleep medicine world, as she stays current and has years of experience treating patients with Narcolepsy. Patients speak highly of her; she truly inspires those around her!

Savanna Osburn, B.S., Osteopathic Medical Student-III,
Lincoln Memorial University-DeBusk College of
Osteopathic Medicine

Dr. Stultz is an inspiration to so many! I have had the privilege to work with her as a medical student, and she puts patient care at the forefront of all she does. She is compassionate, patient, and understanding. Her dedication to research in the field of sleep and Narcolepsy is truly remarkable. She is making a positive difference in the lives of so many patients and their families!

Sylvia Pawlowska-Wajswol, DO, Psychiatry Resident,
Marshall University School of Medicine

Dr . Debra Stultz is the right person for this very significant calling of shining light on the often mysterious and misunderstood condition of Narcolepsy. Dr. Stultz reminds us how excessive daytime sleepiness and cataplexy are often overlooked, dismissed, disparaged, and easily mistaken as other entities. In Wake Up Sleepy Head, she shows us in her unique way how vital it is to make each encounter with a sleepy patient a personalized, detailed, exhaustive, fact-finding, caring, empathic experience. Whether you are a Narcoleptologist, a beginning clinician, or a very sleepy patient, Wake Up Sleepy Head is a clinic on reclaiming the present-day, frequently lost message at the center of patient care—the patient! No one is a more effective teacher and caregiver than Dr. Debra Stultz.

Lewis J. Kass, MD, FAAP
Director of Pediatric Sleep Medicine, Norwalk Hospital
Westchester Pediatric Pulmonology and Sleep Medicine

Dr. Stultz is one of the premier Narcolepsy experts I know, and it is wonderful to have a book highlighting the significant challenges with Narcolepsy! Patients with Narcolepsy and clinicians alike would benefit from this book. I have worked with her on many projects and am very excited to see her work be published like this. This is a must-have!

Asim Roy, MD
Medical Director, Ohio Sleep Medicine Institute

Narcolepsy patients have no greater friend or advocate than Dr. Debra Stultz. I have known Debra for many years, and from her, I have learned a great deal about the compassionate care of individuals struggling with hypersomnolence. I have spoken to Debra about many matters related to Narcolepsy identification, management, and patient care. I have no doubt that any provider who treats patients or patients with narcolepsy will find a wealth of information within these pages.

W. Christopher Winter, MD, D-ABSM, D-ABPN, F-AASM
Sleep Specialist/Neurologist, Author of *The Rested Child*
and *The Sleep Solution*,
Host of Sleep Unplugged with Dr. Chris Winter

Dedication

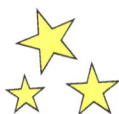

This book is dedicated to my children, family, friends, and work-family, who have supported me tirelessly throughout this journey. I thank you all so very much and love you dearly!

A special thank you to Tyler Burns, MA, LPC, AADC, NCC, for his creative and intellectual support in this book and my many academic adventures!

And to my patients, who have taught me so much about resilience and strength—

You are my heroes!!

In loving memory of

Joseph L. Stultz

Sean Hammack

Glenn Burris, M.D.

Contents

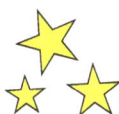

Medications commonly referred to in this book

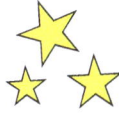

Nuvigil (armodafinil)

Provigil (modafinil)

Wakix (pitolisant)

Sunosi (solriamfetol)

Xyrem (sodium oxybate)

Lumryz (sodium oxybate)

Xywav (calcium, magnesium, potassium & sodium oxybate)

Stimulants

Antidepressants

See Appendix #3 for a complete list of sleep medications, anti-anxiety treatments, stimulants, wake-promoting agents, antidepressants, and mood stabilizers used in treating this disorder.

Introduction

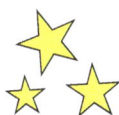

Let's talk about your sleep . . . or rather, your lack thereof . . .

Let's talk about the sleepiness that intrudes into every area of your life.

Let's talk about the muscle weakness occurring with your laughter, anger, or strong emotions.

Let's talk about the isolation you feel when others don't understand.

Let's talk about your options and how you can wake up to your Narcolepsy and a brand new day!!!

Each time I write the word Narcolepsy or even speak it, it is with a capital "N" because I feel so strongly about this disorder and the patients I have treated. I have learned so much from my patients over the years. I have been amazed at their resilience! I authored this book to help patients and their families understand Narcolepsy, how it may impair their lives, and what options they have for change, as well as to help create opportunities to educate those around them about this disorder. It was written as a call to action after I have treated many Narcolepsy patients who do not know where to turn after finally getting an answer for their extended severe excessive daytime sleepiness.

I also hope those who read this book will look for others around them with similar symptoms that may not have been diagnosed or treated yet. What if you could help just one person figure out what is causing their frustrating symptoms? You may even want to look at other members of your family who were always referred to as "sleepy heads," as it can run in families. It is time we all worked together to promote awareness of this disorder.

I have also written this book for primary care providers, sleep physicians, therapists, residents, medical students, and drug reps to help them better understand this disorder and ways to help their patients. I have provided as many resources as possible, including YouTube videos, TED Talk links, pictures, quotes, stories from my patients, etc., to help you grasp all the many ways Narcolepsy can present and the many options for treatment.

I will begin by providing an overall review of the symptoms of Narcolepsy, generalized sleep staging definitions, a brief discussion on how to diagnose Narcolepsy, and general guidelines on how to treat Narcolepsy. Brief discussions on comorbid sleep disorders and how Narcolepsy can look different in different age groups will also be presented.

While this may seem detailed at times, it will help lay the framework for the rest of the book. After you review the information, the other chapters will be much more readable and easier to understand. If it seems too detailed at first, I suggest you look at things out of order. Maybe start with a quick review of Chapter 12 about famous people with Narcolepsy, TV shows that feature Narcolepsy, movies about Narcolepsy, and quotes from my patients about their symptoms. Then perhaps glance at the various presentations of cataplexy in Chapter 2, or even the behavioral treatments of insomnia in Chapter 3, but then come back to this area and start at the beginning as I do believe the Intro and Chapter 1 will provide you the framework of Narcolepsy. I think this will give you a general understanding of this disorder and a progression of all the steps involved in recognizing, diagnosing, treating, and living with Narcolepsy.

Symptoms of Narcolepsy

So, let's start with a definition of Narcolepsy. Narcolepsy consists of periods of **excessive daytime sleepiness (EDS)** and **irresistible urges to sleep** occurring for at least three months **with or without cataplexy**. Cataplexy is any transient muscle weakness associated with emotion.

It is a **lifelong** disorder. Narcolepsy is a **24-hour-a-day disorder**! Let me say that again—it is a 24-hour-a-day disorder with the intrusion of sleep into wakefulness and wake into sleep. The boundaries between sleep and wake are often blurred.

Let's review the primary symptoms associated with Narcolepsy. It usually consists of a variety of symptoms. Unintentionally falling asleep is often called a **"sleep attack"** or "irresistible urge to sleep." **Hypersomnia or excessive daytime sleepiness is the only symptom necessary for diagnosing Narcolepsy, and 100% of patients with Narcolepsy will have this symptom.** Narcolepsy is an instability of the sleep-wake cycle, causing variations during wake, but also disrupted nocturnal sleep, sleep fragmentation, and lighter stages of sleep. Narcolepsy patients may have **"automatic behavior,"** which is the continuation of behavior without memory during microsleeps, where literally "the lights are on, but there is no one at home!" They are physically awake, but their brain is asleep. People with Narcolepsy dream early into sleep, and often, their dreams are so vivid that it is hard for them to distinguish reality and whether they are awake or asleep, which can be almost as intense as a delusion. Also, **insomnia** can be an issue. And some people think you cannot have insomnia if you have Narcolepsy, but that is just not true. Sleep is very fragmented in the Narcolepsy patient.

Narcolepsy is associated with abnormalities of REM sleep activity, resulting in cataplexy, hypnogogic hallucinations, and sleep paralysis.

Cataplexy is any intermittent muscle weakness associated with emotion and occurs when a patient is awake and has an intrusion of REM, causing muscle weakness or even a complete collapse. Cataplexy occurs in roughly 65-75% of patients but may be delayed in presentation or not recognized for several years (Cheung et al., 2017).

Sleep paralysis occurs when someone wakes from REM sleep, and their mind is awake, but their body still has the muscle atonia (paralysis) of REM sleep. They feel as if they cannot move or yell out. Sleep paralysis can occur in anyone with significant sleep deprivation, and there is even a familial type of sleep paralysis without the other symptoms of Narcolepsy. Sleep paralysis can feel very scary, and patients complain of feeling "trapped" in the dream or sleep state. These symptoms have mistakenly been diagnosed as nocturnal panic in some.

Hypnogogic and hypnopompic hallucinations occur when patients experience auditory, visual, sensory, tactile, or other unusual sensations while going to or coming from sleep. It occurs most commonly while going to sleep. Patients can describe this as sensing a presence in the room or as if someone is touching them. They can hear music, hear voices, or see things.

Sleep paralysis occurs in 25–50% of Narcolepsy patients, and hypnogogic/hypnopompic hallucinations occur in 33–80% (Roth et al., 2013).

Disrupted nocturnal sleep occurs. Narcolepsy patients go into REM sleep more quickly; have less NREM slow wave stage 3 NREM sleep (considered a deeper, more restorative state of sleep physically); and have frequent sleep stage changes, all of which lead to disrupted nocturnal sleep and lighter stages of sleep.

Narcolepsy is also often associated with **concentration issues and poor memory ("brain fog")**. Naumann et al. (2006) reported decreased attention and executive functions with Narcolepsy, but memory and routine alertness tasks are either unaffected or only mildly impaired (Naumann, A. et al., 2006). Bayard et al. reported that drug-free patients with Narcolepsy "complained of attention deficit, with altered executive control of attention being explained by the severity of objective sleepiness and global intellectual level" (Bayard, S. et al., 2012). Patients frequently complain of slowed thoughts or difficulty thinking, poor attention skills, and decreased memory and describe this in the following ways:

"As if I am walking through sludge."

"I am missing parts of conversations."

"I can't absorb the details."

"Like the camera is out of focus in my mind."

"My husband swears he tells me things I have not heard."

"Focusing at school is very difficult for me."

"I can't think fast enough."

"I am in a daze . . . a fog at times."

"Sometimes I just cannot complete my work assignments, no matter how hard I try. I am just not thinking right."

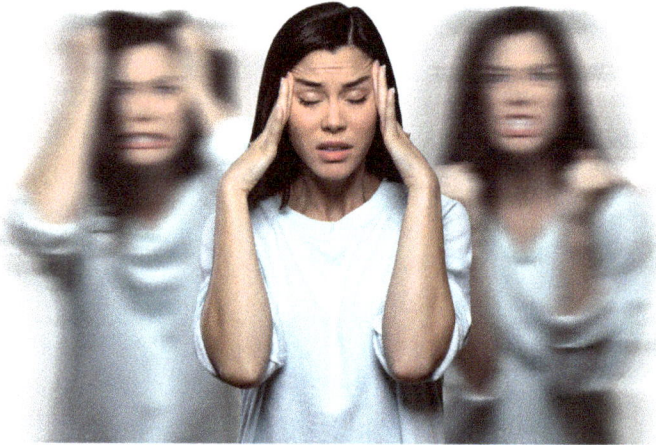

It can start after an acute viral illness, autoimmune illness, head injury, or other neurological disorders and can present with persistent sleepiness and possibly weight gain (especially in children).

The personal impact of Narcolepsy can be widespread for the patient and their life. Sometimes the changes come on so gradually, patients do not even realize they have made significant accommodations over the years to cope with the illness. Family members and friends also have to adjust their schedules and expectations when there is a person with Narcolepsy. This point was demonstrated by Thorpy et al. (M. J. Thorpy, et al., 2019), who indicated that "the vast majority of physicians (93.6%) noted that people with Narcolepsy unknowingly alter their lives to accommodate their symptoms;

a much smaller percentage of patients (40%) reported avoiding social situations, and 20% reported avoiding strong emotions." Often, this can lead to isolation, impaired social relationships, impaired emotional development, and not reaching full academic or occupational achievement.

A mnemonic frequently used to describe Narcolepsy and to help remember all of the five possible symptoms that may be present is **CHESS** (Pelayo R, 2006), which stands for:

Cataplexy

Hypnogogic/**H**ypnopompic **H**allucinations

Excessive daytime sleepiness

Sleep paralysis

Sleep disruptions.

The symptoms of Narcolepsy vary from person to person and may change over time. The symptoms may look different in the pediatric case compared to the adult case and can even appear different in the elderly. Narcolepsy in pediatric patients may present with irritability, hyperactivity, behavioral problems, complex movements, and facial grimacing. You may also see the resumption of naps or longer sleep over 24 hours. Although cataplexy may be present in the pediatric patient, it may not start or be recognized/diagnosed until much later. The presentation of cataplexy in children can involve having more slurred speech and weakness in the face or what looks like muscle twitching or tics, with adolescents having more weakness in the limbs. The frequency and severity of cataplexy attacks may be higher for pediatric patients.

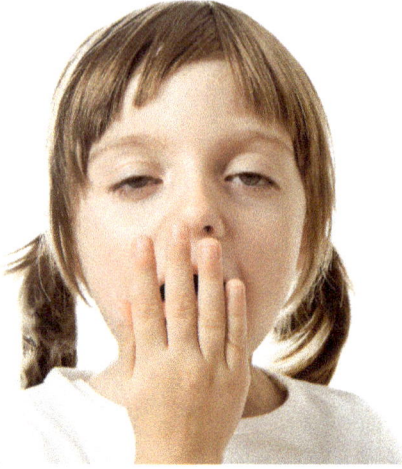

The presentation of Narcolepsy at the age of diagnosis has been reported to look different before and after 18 years of age by Zhang and associates (M. Zhang et al., 2020), who observed children had increased obesity, night eating, parasomnias, ADHD, sleep-talking, and sleep drunkenness. The adult patients had decreased quality of life findings and increased apnea events. Pediatric Narcolepsy is discussed in more detail in Chapter 6. We need to realize that Narcolepsy can be present in the younger population, and we should consider it a possible diagnosis in all kids with sleepiness, academic difficulty, irritability, etc.

When Narcolepsy starts in childhood or adolescence, the diagnosis may be delayed for many years after the onset of hypersomnia, with Dauvilliers et al. (2001) reporting two onset peaks, the first occurring around 14.7 years old and the second around 35 years of age. Frauscher and associates (Frauscher et al., 2013) found that, on average, it took patients 6.5 years to be diagnosed with Narcolepsy after their first symptom, with most being diagnosed with something else first. Newer studies suggest this time may be shortening, and there is much we can do to help prevent this delay!

Although Narcolepsy usually presents much earlier in life, "Late-life Narcolepsy" is often significantly overlooked as a possibility in older adults. It could be because the patient had symptoms that may not have been recognized for years, or it could be a new onset and possibly secondary to another disorder (such as neurologic disorders). It was reported (Chakravorty & Rye, 2003) that elderly patients with Narcolepsy may be less sleepy and less likely to have the other REM-related abnormalities of this disorder. They suggested Narcoleptic patients may tend to adjust their lifestyle more towards self-employment based on their sleepiness. Also, significant morbidity can occur due to cataplexy falls in older adults and even with the extensive work-up for cataplexy itself. They described exacerbation of Narcolepsy/cataplexy due to concurrent medical disorders (such as diabetes and sleep apnea) and lab abnormalities. Sleepiness in the elderly can present in multiple ways and is often confused with medication side effects, medication overuse, other neurologic or psychiatric symptoms, depression, grief, or apathy.

The older patient with Narcolepsy may have increased comorbidities of other sleep disorders besides their Narcolepsy, such as obstructive sleep apnea, severe restless legs syndrome, and periodic limb movement disorder. If present, all these disorders need to be aggressively treated simultaneously. Sleepiness is often dismissed in older adults as an expected age-related change. Cataplexy can still be significant in the elderly but is often the reason for an extensive medical work-up to identify the cause. Narcolepsy may not even be anywhere in the differential diagnosis considered in this age group. Secondary Narcolepsy may be associated with disorders such as demyelinating diseases like

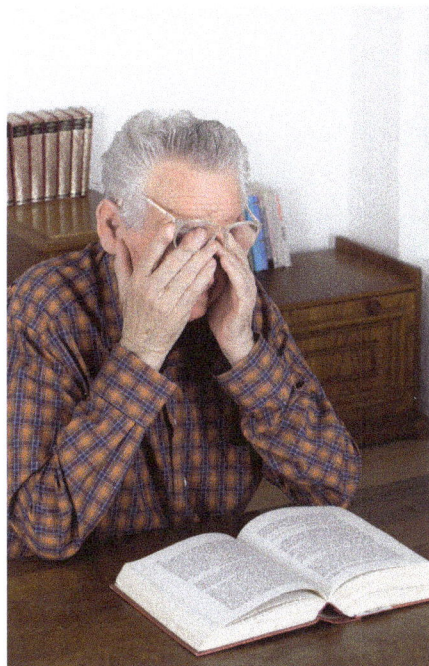

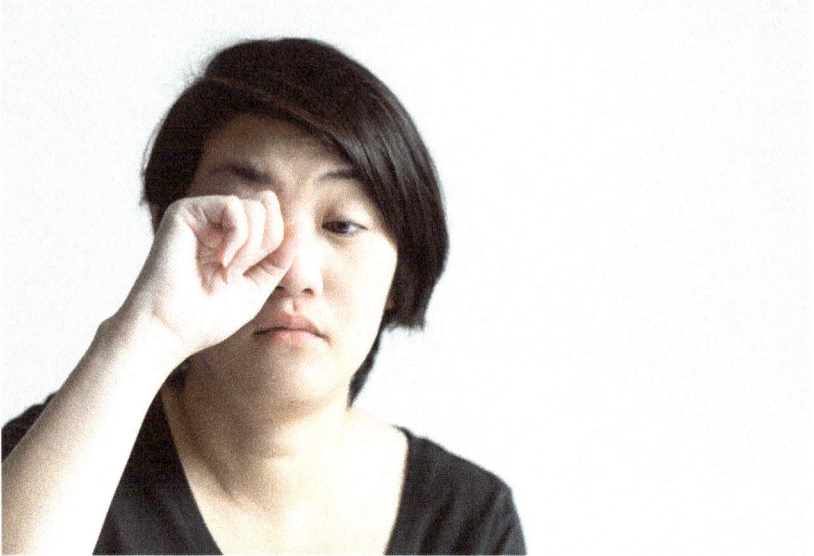

Multiple Sclerosis (MS), Parkinson's, Alzheimer's, head injuries, tumors, CVAs (cerebral vascular accidents or strokes), sarcoidosis, paraneoplastic conditions, and various illnesses more common in the elderly.

There may also be differences in presentation in males vs. females, as females have more hormonal changes that could contribute to sleepiness. Won et al. 2014 suggested women had a delay in diagnosis and had more objective sleepiness on the MSLT sleep test used to diagnose Narcolepsy. Females may have more cataplexy, and there may be a longer delay in diagnosis for them. Females may also have more severe symptoms but underestimate their severity. Men often have more complaints of sleepiness and mainly focus on occupational impairments from this symptom. More studies are needed to address the differences between the sexes, but their presentation generally is similar.

Definition of Narcolepsy

In *The AASM International Classification of Sleep Disorders* book (*International Classification of Sleep Disorders*, 2014), Narcolepsy is classified as type 1 or 2 based on the presence or absence of cataplexy and/or decreased cerebral spinal fluid (CSF) hypocretin-1 levels. (Lumbar puncture CSF evaluation is not necessary for diagnosing Narcolepsy and aids primarily in diagnostic clarification and research arenas.) They also report a low familial prevalence of 1% to 2% risk that first-degree relatives of Narcolepsy patients will have the disorder, but this is a significant increase over the risk in the general population.

Types of Sleep

Before we go on, we need to talk about the distinct types of sleep. Our sleep consists of REM sleep (rapid eye movement) and NREM or non-REM sleep. During REM sleep, our brain is highly active, and our body is usually paralyzed. During non-REM sleep (NREM), we have three stages of sleep, with lighter sleep occurring during stage 1 and deeper sleep occurring in stage 3 NREM sleep. We believe stage 3 NREM sleep is a deeper, more restorative stage of sleep physically. Narcolepsy patients fall asleep quickly, go into REM sleep fast, and have frequent arousals at night. They have disruption of their REM sleep, best described as a flickering of REM sleep both during the daytime and at night, leading to cataplexy, sleep paralysis, hypnogogic hallucinations, vivid dreams, and nightmares. They have light fragmented NREM sleep with frequent stage switches and disruptions, which limits their amount of stage 3 NREM sleep.

Disorders Comorbid with Narcolepsy

Narcolepsy is associated with a variety of comorbid disorders. Black et al. (2017) and Ohayon (Ohayon, 2013) reported a higher risk in patients with Narcolepsy of:

- 2.1 times increased heart disease
- 1.3 times increased risk of hypertension
- 1.8 times increased risk of diabetes
- 1.5 times increased hypercholesterolemia
- 2.5 times increased risk of stroke
- 2.3 times the risk of obesity.

Weight gain can occur around the onset of Narcolepsy. Increased weight can occur in both pediatric and adult populations and may quickly increase in children. Precocious puberty may occur in 17% of pediatric Narcolepsy patients, compared to 1.9% of the general pediatric obese population (Quaedackers et al., 2021). Precocious puberty is puberty changes beginning before age 8 in girls and before the age of 9 in boys, causing changes in body shape and size, the rapid growth of bones and muscles, and the ability to reproduce. Maski and associates (2017) reported increased mental fogginess; difficulty thinking, remembering, concentrating, or paying attention; irritability; and mood instability with Narcolepsy. Maski also reported weight gain in 16.3% of those having Narcolepsy with cataplexy and 14.7% without cataplexy.

Comorbid psychiatric disorders such as depression, bipolar, and anxiety (social anxiety, panic, and agoraphobia) are common (Ohayon, 2013), as is the comorbidity of other sleep disorders such as obstructive sleep apnea (Sansa et al., 2010), REM sleep behavior disorder (Nightingale et al., 2005), and Periodic Limb Movement Disorder (Pereira et al., 2014).

Let me explain these other sleep disorders in a little more detail. Narcolepsy can co-exist with sleep apnea, with 5-6% of those with **Obstructive Sleep Apnea (OSA)** having Narcolepsy and a more significant percentage of those with Narcolepsy also having OSA. OSA patients snore, have obstructive airways, and complain of excessive daytime sleepiness. **Periodic Limb Movement Disorder (PLMD)** is the repetitive twitching or jerking of the legs or arms/hands during sleep that disrupts sleep, leading to fragmentation of the sleep stages and lighter stages of sleep, which causes daytime sleepiness. **Restless Legs Syndrome (RLS)** is an unusual sensation causing the desire to move, rub, or stretch the legs or arms. Restless Legs Syndrome occurs before sleep or during periods of wakefulness. Periodic Limb Movement Disorder, by definition, occurs only during sleep. RLS and PLMD are sometimes associated but are not the same. **REM Sleep Behavior Disorder (RBD)** is a sleep disorder in which patients act out their dreams. Usually, during REM sleep, the brain is highly active, but the muscles are paralyzed. With REM Behavior Disorder, there is an "unhooking" of the paralysis, and patients may punch out, kick, yell out, or even get out of bed acting out whatever they are dreaming about.

Narcolepsy can also be associated with head injuries. Sleepiness can occur acutely and or chronically after a head injury. Chronic hypersomnia may be overlooked as associated with a head injury or concussion. Sandsmark and associates (Sandsmark et al., 2017) reported excessive daytime sleepiness, nighttime sleep fragmentation, and insomnia have been found in adult and pediatric populations, as well as in animal studies after different forms of traumatic brain injury, which may persist for years. They reported patients might have pleiosomnia (an increased need for sleep), requiring an additional 1–2 hours of sleep per 24-hour cycle.

A study by Lankford and associates (Lankford et al., 1994) indicated that "Narcolepsy may be 'dormant' and that, in cases genetically at risk, even a minor injury to the central nervous system can cause that person to become symptomatic." With the above in mind, our group did a retrospective review of patients with a prior diagnosis of Narcolepsy and found that 28% had a history of a head injury of varying severity (Stultz et al., 2021).

Diagnosing Narcolepsy

To diagnose Narcolepsy, we use a detailed sleep history and sleep studies. Two distinct types of sleep studies are involved. An overnight sleep study is called a polysomnogram (PSG) (Deak & Epstein, 2009). The second type of study needed is called a Multiple Sleep Latency Test (MSLT) (Carskadon, 1986a) or nap study, in which the patient is given up to five opportunities to fall asleep, and we measure how quickly they go to sleep, if they have REM sleep, and, if so, how fast they go into REM sleep. I will explain these tests in greater detail in Chapter 4.

The Narcolepsy Network (www.narcolepsynetwork.org) reports Narcolepsy affects 3 million people worldwide, or 0.04% of people worldwide. Based on a U.S. 2010–2019 consensus study and an article by Scammel (Scammell, 2015), Narcolepsy is estimated to occur in about 165,000–200,000 people in the United States—however, as this disorder often goes undiagnosed, it is likely much higher. A YouTube video called "What is Narcolepsy?" by Harvard Medical School shows Dr. Scammell giving a good description of Narcolepsy and what areas of the brain we feel are involved in this disorder.

A recent study reported that the overall annual incidence (which is the occurrence of new cases over a period of time) per 100,000/year was 7.67 for overall Narcolepsy, 7.13 without cataplexy, and 4.87 with cataplexy (Scheer et al., 2019). This study also revealed an increase in females, those without cataplexy, those aged 21–30, and those residing in the north-central region of the United States. Acquavella et al. (2020) reported the prevalence (the proportion of a population with a specific disease) of Narcolepsy per 100,000 patients rose by 14% from 2013 to 2016. Since then, there have been rapid advancements in sleep medicine, specifically for Narcolepsy, so I feel it is likely even more prevalent.

The Nexus Narcolepsy Registry (Ohayon et al., 2021) reports that Narcolepsy is often misdiagnosed, commonly occurs during childhood or adolescence, and takes many years and multiple consults to get the correct diagnosis. Those who had symptoms starting in childhood often had longer delays in diagnosis. It has been suggested that it is as common as multiple sclerosis or Parkinson's, and we all know people with these disorders. I bet you know other people with Narcolepsy too!

Treatment of Narcolepsy

Narcolepsy can be dangerous if sleep or cataplexy occurs while driving, walking downstairs, or in other hazardous situations. Narcolepsy is associated with increased accidents and increased use of health care expenses. Thankfully, many treatment options are becoming available.

In this book, I will outline different medications and behavioral treatments found to be helpful for Narcolepsy. We are fortunate as many new medications are on the horizon for treatment in this field! In Appendix 3, at the end of the book, I have provided a list of frequently used medications to treat Narcolepsy and its associated disorders in their brand and generic names to assist you in discovering treatment options. I have also listed medicines for depression and anxiety, some of which can interfere with your MSLT test. Many people with Narcolepsy have co-existing depression and anxiety and will need some of these meds. A helpful suggestion would be to keep a list of all the medications you have tried previously and the ones you are currently taking to share with your current or future providers. (Use the list provided in Appendix #3 to do that.) Keep an eye out for new treatment options listed on Narcolepsy websites and the internet, and adjust your treatment plan as alternatives become available.

Throughout this book, I hope to give you examples from my patients or my readings to help you understand how subtle, brief, or dramatic the presentations of Narcolepsy may be. Knowledge is power; the more we make others aware of this disease, the faster it can be diagnosed and treated appropriately. Our job—mine and yours—is to educate your family, friends, primary care provider, sleep physician, employer, community, the kids and teachers at school, college-aged students, and those with a history of a head injury. You get the point. Let's spread the word!

Now, let's look more specifically into the symptoms of Narcolepsy. May I suggest you first read this book while highlighting things of interest.

Then, using the table at the back of the book:

- list the top 10 things you learned from it
- the top 5 people you want to share it with, and then
- develop an action plan of 5 specific things you want to initiate immediately.

Chapter 1

"Help . . . I'm Sleepy, and I Can't Get Up!"

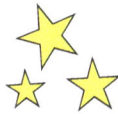

⭐⭐

Understanding the Symptoms and Potential Causes of Narcolepsy and Hypersomnia

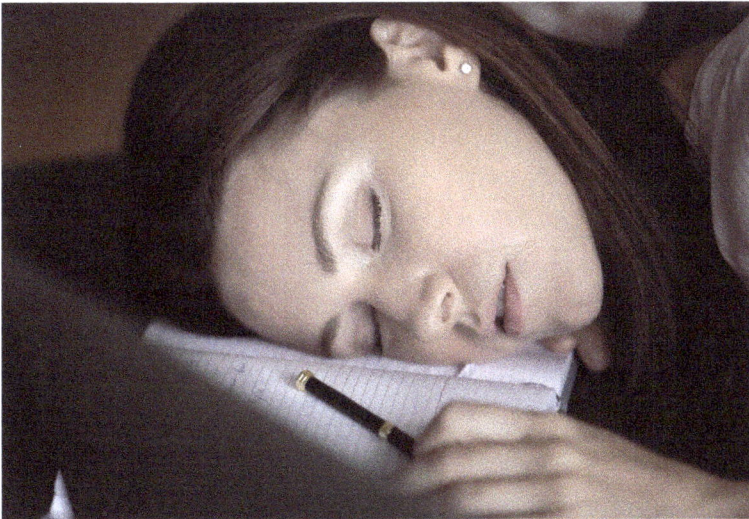

"I'm awake . . . I'm asleep . . . I am waking up during my sleep . . .
I am falling asleep while I am awake!"
Anonymous patient from my office

The International Classification of Sleep Disorders 3rd Edition (American Academy of Sleep Medicine, 2014) defines excessive daytime sleepiness (EDS) or hypersomnia as "the inability to maintain alertness or wakefulness with unintentionally falling asleep almost daily for at least three months" (as opposed to fatigue with a lack of physical or mental energy). The differential diagnosis in a patient presenting with excessive daytime sleepiness includes Narcolepsy, poor sleep hygiene, not allowing enough time to sleep, shift work, psychiatric disorders (anxiety, depression, PTSD), a sleep environment with pets or kids in the bed, hormonal issues, hot flashes, various prescription or over the counter medications, substance abuse, other sleep disorders such as OSA, RLS, PLMD, and other medical diseases (Parkinson's, traumatic brain injury, MS, tumors). Chronic pain is also a significant cause of sleep disruption, poor-quality sleep, and complaints of hypersomnia. And the list goes on.

Another diagnosis similar to Narcolepsy and which must be ruled out is **Idiopathic Hypersomnia (IH)**. This diagnosis requires a history of daily sleepiness of at least three months duration, where there has been sufficient time to sleep, in a patient with a mean sleep onset latency of less than or equal to eight minutes on the MSLT (nap study), greater than or equal to 660 minutes of sleep (usually 12–14 hours), fewer than two sleep onset REM periods on the MSLT, and the absence of cataplexy. Increased awareness and attention to IH resurfaced with the approval of Xywav (calcium, magnesium, potassium, and sodium oxybates) and the recent orphan drug status for Wakix (pitilosant) use for treating this disorder.

For the diagnosis of IH, Narcolepsy must be excluded. Patients with IH can have other associated features such as headaches, syncope, orthostatic hypotension, and peripheral vascular complaints like Raynaud's syndrome, (which may cause the patients' fingers to turn pale or white, then blue and even flushed with stress or exposure to the cold). Impaired body temperature sensitivity and regulation also occur in some patients with Idiopathic Hypersomnia who are sometimes too cold or feverish. IH patients can also have sleep inertia or "sleep drunkenness." They can be exhausted by loud noise, extreme heat, or extreme emotional events. So, as you can see, this diagnosis is close to that of Narcolepsy; however, there is no cataplexy, and the patient must not meet the Narcolepsy criteria of two sleep onset REM periods on their MSLT examination.

"Even where sleep is concerned, too much is a bad thing."

Homer

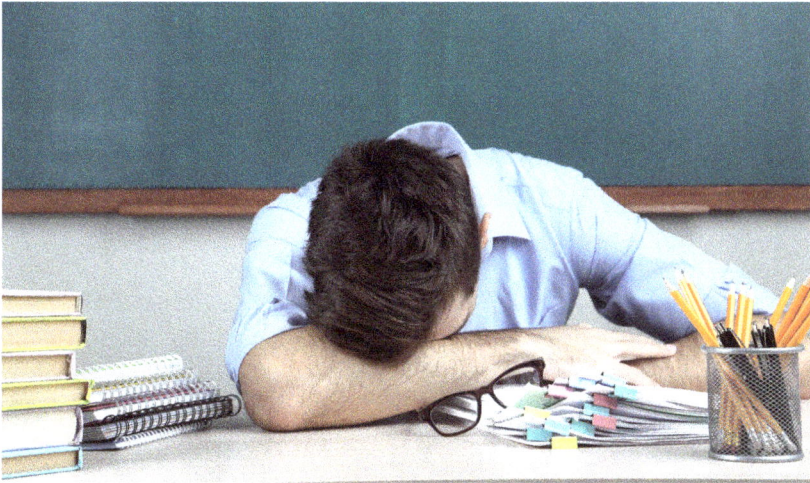

So, the first step in evaluating EDS or hypersomnia is to look around at all the possible contributing factors and realize it may be more than just one thing. Narcolepsy, however, should always be on that list of possible explanations.

There are two ways to diagnose Narcolepsy, one using *The International Classification of Sleep Disorders* (ICSD) criteria and the other way using the *Diagnostic and Statistical Manual of Mental Disorders 5th Edition* (American Psychiatric Association, 2013) (DSM-V) criteria. We will discuss this in greater detail in Chapter 4, including the complete steps to diagnose Narcolepsy, but I will outline the differences between the ICSD-3 and the DSM-V below:

ICSD Diagnostic Criteria (Both A and B must be met.)
A. The patient has **daily** periods of irrepressible need to sleep or daytime lapses into sleep occurring for **at least three months**.
B. The presence of **one or both** of the following:
    a. Cataplexy and a mean sleep onset latency of less than eight minutes, in addition to two or more sleep onset REM periods (SOREMP). A SOREMP is defined as when REM sleep occurs within the first fifteen minutes of sleep onset during an MSLT performed according to standard techniques. A sleep onset REM period (SOREMP) within fifteen minutes of sleep onset on the preceding overnight nocturnal polysomnogram may replace one of the SOREMPs on the MSLT.
    b. Cerebrospinal fluid (CSF) obtained from a lumbar puncture reveals a hypocretin-1 concentration of less than or equal to 110 pg/mL or less than 1/3 of mean values obtained in normal subjects with the same standardized assay.

DSM-V Diagnostic Criteria
A. Recurrent periods of an irrepressible need to sleep, lapses into sleep, or napping occurring within the same day. These must have happened **at least three times per week** over the past **three months**.
B. The presence of **at least one** of the following:
    a. Episodes of cataplexy, occurring at least a few times per month, defined as either of the below:
        1) In individuals with long-standing disease, brief (seconds to minutes) episodes of

sudden bilateral loss of muscle tone with maintained consciousness are precipitated by emotions such as laughter or joking.

2) In children or individuals within six months of onset, spontaneous grimaces, or jaw-opening episodes with tongue thrusting or global hypotonia, without any obvious emotional triggers.

b. A hypocretin deficiency is measured using cerebrospinal fluid (CSF). Low CSF levels of hypocretin-1 must not be observed in the context of acute brain injury, inflammation, or infection.

c. Nocturnal sleep polysomnography (PSG) shows a rapid eye movement (REM) sleep onset latency less than or equal to fifteen minutes, or a multiple sleep latency test showing a mean sleep latency less than or equal to eight minutes and two or more sleep-onset REM periods.

As you can see, these criteria are similar, but one main difference is that the Multiple Sleep Latency Test (MSLT) is one of the ways Narcolepsy is diagnosed in the ICSD and is not absolutely necessary for the diagnosis of Narcolepsy using the DSM-V criteria if the patient has either cataplexy or CSF hypocretin abnormalities. A lumbar puncture with CSF evaluation is not routinely required for the diagnosis but may be helpful for diagnostic clarification or research purposes.

As stated previously, one huge misconception is that people with Narcolepsy could not possibly have insomnia. Nothing could be further from the truth! Their sleep is fragmented, with intrusions of wakefulness during sleep, vivid dreams, and other sleep disorder symptoms. This book has a whole chapter on insomnia and disrupted nocturnal sleep in Narcolepsy.

The quote at the beginning of the chapter is so accurate. There are intrusions of sleep into wakefulness and wake during sleep, like a light switch flickering. So, everything is off in most Narcolepsy patients . . . and remember, it is a 24-hour-a-day illness! Let's now talk about other clarifications and associations for this disorder.

Types of Narcolepsy

There are two types of Narcolepsy: type 1 with cataplexy and type 2 without cataplexy. As mentioned, the only symptom you must have to be diagnosed with Narcolepsy is excessive daytime sleepiness, and the presence or absence of cataplexy distinguishes type 1 from type 2. We will explore cataplexy and its various presentations in Chapter 2.

We do not always know what starts Narcolepsy, which is primarily idiopathic (an illness that arises spontaneously without a known cause). Still, there are cases of secondary Narcolepsy arising due to various factors. It may be genetic, especially with younger onset, and it is thought that up to 30% may be related to a specific trigger event such as head trauma, stroke, strep infection, mononucleosis (mono), H1N1, and heavy metal exposure. And what about post-COVID? What about the "long haulers" from COVID? Who knows ?? Narcolepsy symptoms may be on the rise after COVID too. It may be a one-two punch with susceptible individuals having a trigger.

As discussed earlier, secondary Narcolepsy can occur after a head injury, and there is a three-to-four-time risk increase after a motor vehicle accident. Patients may not realize the consequences of a head injury when they fell off the monkey bars as a kid, hit their head on the windshield during a motor vehicle accident, took a hit to their head with a baseball during the game, had repeated concussions playing football, or with military blast injuries, and falls, and so on. It is potentially associated with strep, Lyme disease, mono, influenza, brain tumors, vascular disease, and the H1N1 vaccine in Europe. Cases have also been reported with other neurologic conditions such as MS, Parkinson's, hypothalamic tumors, encephalitis, Prader-Willi Syndrome, Alzheimer's, and myotonic dystrophy. I have had two patients who were sisters with myotonic dystrophy, both having Narcolepsy.

For many years, I have been fascinated by this disorder and the strength of character of those with Narcolepsy. The years of sleepiness and struggles for answers, support, and understanding is a difficult journey few will ever grasp. Sleepiness, while overwhelming, may gradually appear until it becomes the norm and may be accepted as an internal weakness of drive or determination. Patients may then be labeled lazy, unmotivated, uncaring, or depressed. The struggles create personal, academic, occupational, and professional issues. Suffering in silence and isolation while searching for answers and directions from someone with a bit of knowledge to help them is often very difficult. All these things lead to the patient feeling discouraged and often depressed and out of control. Sleep is ruling their life.

Fighting to stay awake creates what I like to call "The Pressure Cooker of Sleepiness," with irresistible urges to sleep, where sleepiness builds like the top pressure cooker regulator or "jiggler" of a pressure cooker until there is no control over the drive for sleep. Sleep takes over.

People use many words to describe sleepiness and may not even use the word sleepy. They may say, "I'm tired." And there are various kinds of tired. Patients may have "clinomania," a powerful urge to stay in bed without sleeping for extended periods. Hanging out in bed does not help with sleepiness and can be counterproductive. It can cause your brain to not associate your bed with sleep. Excessive daytime sleepiness can present as irritability or even hyperactivity in an effort to stay awake (this is especially true in children). It can be misdiagnosed as ADHD, depression, laziness, or apathy. Narcolepsy can interfere with school, work, family relationships, and emotional and social development.

"Sometimes before bedtime, I fall asleep on the couch; it's my little sleep appetizer. My Nappetizer."

Narcolepsy patient, Facebook

Once again, sleepiness does not always look sleepy. Narcolepsy patients can present with hyperactivity, irritability, moodiness, fogginess, drooping eyelids, fidgetiness, increased yawning, and nodding off to sleep in the middle of things. One of my patients described a sleep attack as "It's like going from being sober to drunk in three minutes."

I once had a patient who fell asleep while using a jackhammer! Now that is sleepy! But he was so used to working every day with some degree of sleepiness that it did not seem over-alarming. Patients with Narcolepsy may have been called a "sleepyhead" for years and may have built up a tolerance for their degree of sleepiness. Various descriptions of Narcolepsy have been used. Below are a few ways patients have described excessive sleepiness; a more detailed list will be presented in Chapter 12.

"I can't get up in the morning."

"I just can't stay awake."

"I fall asleep unintentionally."

"I must always stay busy to just not fall asleep."

"It's like I am attached to the couch."

"I can't focus."

"I'm a slug."

"I get sleepy when I'm driving. I have had accidents and fender benders."

"I am groggy."

"I was constantly mistaken for drunk."

"I can fall asleep in the middle of anything . . . talking . . . sex."

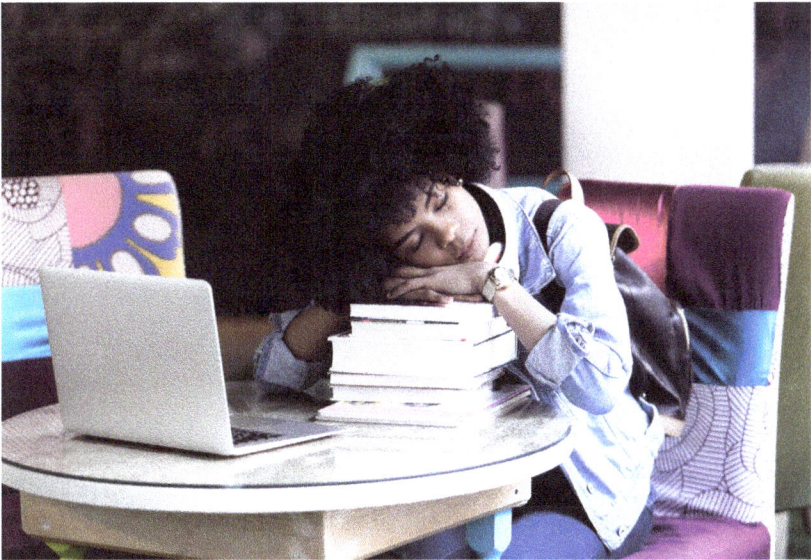

"I am a sloth—cute but sleepy."

"I can't hold my eyes open."

"Drowsy."

"Sluggish."

"Lethargic."

"Slow-moving."

"Asleep on the job."

"Lifeless."

"Disengaged."

"Dead to the world."

"Out of it."

"Half-asleep."

"Sleeping Beauty."

"I catnap a lot."

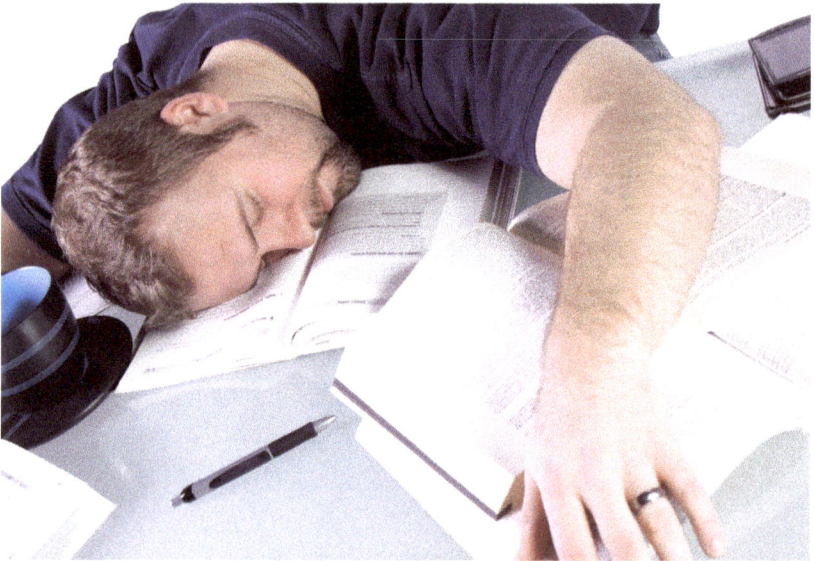

You can look up many examples of sleepy babies and children that may demonstrate REM sleep intrusions, sudden sleep, or extreme drowsiness in YouTube videos. When babies do it, we think it is cute and funny. When adults do it, others believe they are drugged, weird, or "psycho." We will discuss this in greater detail in Chapter 4. For now, you can try looking up the following YouTube videos:

- Funny babies and kids who are falling asleep in awkward situations: https://youtu.be/uL_CEZbeC_0
- Funny cute baby falling asleep standing up: https://youtu.be/yqd_9p546Ts
- Funny babies can fall asleep in every situation compilation 2017: https://youtu.be/w_c3wjzctr4

These videos show the sleepiness and the head bobbing of going to sleep with muscle weakness, which is not abnormal in infants and young children who developmentally normally have lots of REM sleep and go quickly into REM. This we outgrow.

It can also occur in dogs. If you are a pet lover, check out Narcolepsy in Dogs on YouTube.

- A Narcoleptic puppy falls asleep when he gets too excited: https://youtu.be/gOvzM8PXkw8
- Narcoleptic dog: https://youtu.be/XOh2nleWTwl
- Snoozy: https://youtu.be/HOkckq9pfoE
- Narcoleptic dogs: https://youtu.be/jTj3a2nHw8k
- Skeeter the Narcoleptic poodle: https://youtu.be/LbmbQkX7czo

You can also search for people with cataplexy and people with Narcolepsy. These are just a few of the videos discussing or demonstrating Narcolepsy:

- Narcoleptic personal trainer documents condition: https://youtu.be/wTQ_SR_BBqs
- What is Narcolepsy: https://youtu.be/Ucpf_OYvs4E
- What is Cataplexy? Julie Flygare Narcolepsy Awareness Video 4 (HD): https://youtu.be/AOA1bJH_d9s
- Medical Stories—Narcolepsy: Carol's Story: https://youtu.be/bpvSk7m5Aw4

- Michael J. Thorpy, MBChB: The Subtle Manifestations of Cataplexy: https://youtu.be/Sar69OuA92U

For now, that's enough about sleepiness—let's move on to the descriptions of cataplexy.

"The feeling of sleepiness when you are not in bed and can't get there, is the meanest feeling in the world."

Edgar Watson Howe

Chapter 2

"You Make Me Weak in the Knees!"

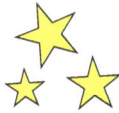

Cataplexy and Its Many Presentations

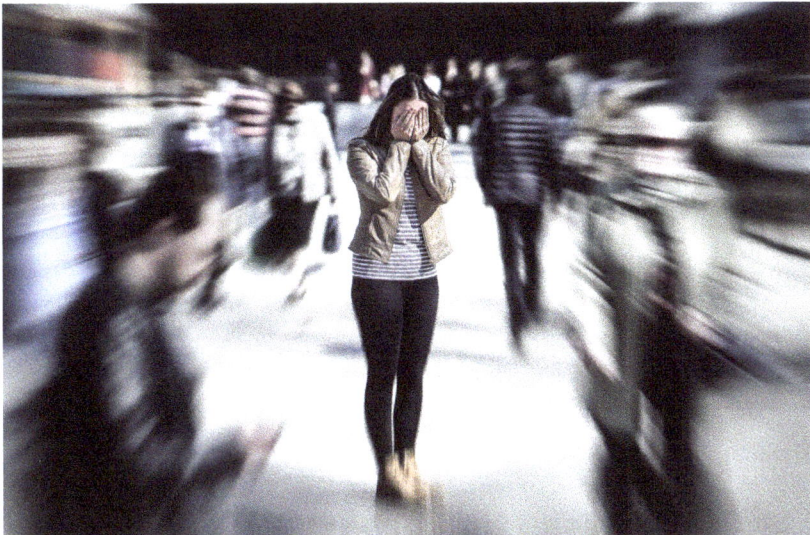

*"Cataplexy: When you're filled with emotions yet lack
the strength to create a physical reaction."*
Unknown, Pinterest

Cataplexy is muscle weakness that occurs suddenly, is temporary, and is precipitated by emotion. Patients are aware during these episodes! They can hear and understand what you say but usually cannot respond. They are still breathing. They still can move their eyes, although their eyes may be closed. Raise their eyelids and look. This may be a way to identify that this is cataplexy and not something else. Alternatively, they may be unaware they even have cataplexy episodes, especially when brief and when they only involve the face or clumsiness. So, checking with a family member or friend about these symptoms is always a good idea.

Cataplexy is an emotionally induced muscle weakness, not a weakness of emotion! It comes from the Latin word *cataplessa*, which means "to strike down with fear or the like." (http://scholarpedia.org/article/ Cataplexy). Other synonyms include strike fear into, freeze, paralyze, scare stiff, stupefy, scare to death, shock, and spook. It can be a subtle, partial, or complete loss of muscle tone and is any muscle weakness associated with an emotion. It can vary from one or two episodes a year to several daily. It is usually transient and resolves spontaneously. Rarely, a patient may have "status cataplecticus," which is the occurrence of prolonged cataplexy over many hours or days without an emotional trigger. This has been reported after the abrupt discontinuation of venlafaxine (Wang & Greenberg, 2013), duloxetine (Hamid et al., 2020), clomipramine (Martínez-Rodríguez et al., 2002), or other antidepressants.

Antidepressants suppress cataplexy. When they are abruptly stopped (especially the shorter-acting ones and the SNRI antidepressants), they can cause rebound cataplexy. This may occur in people who did not even know they have cataplexy if the antidepressants have been used for depression/anxiety for an extended time. Instead, it is often attributed to a withdrawal syndrome from the antidepressant. Additionally, the antidepressant can interfere with the MSLT testing results when trying to diagnose Narcolepsy.

Cataplexy presentation may change over time in the same person—it can look different in the pediatric population versus the adult population, present differently in older adults, and look different with various emotions. It is a symptom specific to Narcolepsy.

A study by Pizza and associates (2018) indicated the involvement of muscles of the head or neck has a high diagnostic accuracy for Narcolepsy, with ptosis (drooping of the upper eyelid), mouth opening, tongue protrusion, head drop, abrupt cessation of smile/facial expression, facial jerks, and grimacing associated with an emotional trigger are descriptive of Narcolepsy. The ICSD-3 definition includes the loss of muscle tone with retained consciousness. Cataplexy occurs in 60–70% of Narcolepsy patients and is pathognomonic (or indicative) of Narcolepsy.

Cataplexy is **not** required for the diagnosis of Narcolepsy. It does not have to be dramatic, but it can be dramatic, with complete collapse. It often presents six or seven years (or longer) after the onset of excessive daytime sleepiness, or at least it is not recognized for several years after the beginning of severe excessive daytime sleepiness. It may be suppressed by antidepressants, making this symptom even more challenging to diagnose in those who may have been on antidepressants for years for depression, anxiety, chronic pain, or migraines. It may be vague and more evident to others than the patients themselves. They may have become so accustomed to this sensation that they do not realize it is not normal.

It can be so brief that the patient is not even sure if something happened or not. Family members may notice the facial grimacing, unevenness of their smile, momentary loss of muscle tone, clumsiness, etc. Family members and friends have been noted to say, "Did you see that?" when they see the brief muscle weakness in the patient's face, hands, or knees, and the patient can be completely unaware of what they are talking about. These episodes can be more severe under significant stress, causing others sometimes to suggest that the cataplexy is due to substance abuse or is of psychiatric origin.

The REM Runner

Julie Flygare, the "Wanjira" (the Kenyan name given to her meaning "a leader"), the "REM Runner," is a patient with Narcolepsy who is a pioneer in the field of sleep medicine and has carried the torch for Narcolepsy for many years. Through her book, *Wide Awake and Dreaming: A Memoir of Narcolepsy* (Flygare, 2012), her lectures, internet posts, involvement in support groups, and more, she has been highly influential in the education about Narcolepsy over the years. She is the President & CEO of Project Sleep, has given a highly informative TEDx Talk, and hosts the Project Sleep podcast. In her book, she provides compelling descriptions of cataplexy and excessive daytime sleepiness during her struggles to complete law school while she developed, was diagnosed, and treated for Narcolepsy. With her descriptions of the melting of her knees with laughter, buckling of her knees with irritation, and the descriptions of cataplexy with sexual activity (which we will discuss more in Chapter 9), she gives an amazing look into the clinical presentations of this disorder. Insights from her story are frequently quoted within this book, and I strongly suggest you consider reading it if you have not already done so. I have recommended it to many patients and recently reread it in preparation for writing this book.

In Chapter 3, when she thought a car would not stop while she was crossing the street and again while watching a *Saturday Night Live* skit, she reported, "My legs turned to Jell-O." In another description of cataplexy, she described head bobbing as, "Tingling in my head came quickly, and my neck gave out, dipping toward my chest, lifting up briefly, then dipping forward again. Just a moment later, my head regained strength." In another description of hand weakness, she revealed, "When someone said something funny, my head tingled, and my hand relaxed its grip on the cup sliding through my fingers. I regained control in time to catch the cup before it fell to the floor. To my friends, my fumble appeared nothing more than momentary clumsiness."

Cataplexy can look like clumsiness, and patients have reported falls, tripping over things, dropping things, and even significant injuries or wrecks secondary to cataplexy. Often, there is some awareness that it is coming (which also may occur with fainting or "passing out"), so patients may be able to sit or collapse away from an object or in a way that would prevent a severe injury. Because of this, many have misdiagnosed this symptom as psychogenic, and the diagnosis may have been delayed even longer. This could not be further from the truth! The differential diagnosis of unusual presentations such as this would include hypotension, transient ischemic attacks, drop attacks, akinetic seizures, muscular disorders, vestibular disorders, psychiatric disorders, pseudo seizures, conversion disorder, neuromuscular disorders, fainting, and malingering, to name a few.

Once again, patients may not even realize they have this symptom. Their family members or friends may be able to describe their cataplexy more accurately. Often, those around them may describe their symptoms in a casual comment such as:

"That thing you do when you laugh."

"Your face looks different when you are telling a funny story."

"Sometimes your eyes look suddenly sleepy when you are describing something."

"Your head almost fell on the plate when you were talking about that."

"Your speech slurs sometimes."

"Did you know you stutter?"

"Remember how we used to make you laugh so
we could see you fall to the ground?"

Having families use cell phones to document cataplexy or any other unusual behavior can be extremely helpful. I once had a patient and her husband describe what sounded like a very extended period of cataplexy, and the more I asked, he said, "I have a video." The video was invaluable in making the diagnosis. The patient could describe everything around her but had complete muscle collapse while sitting (or slumping) on a porch swing, which brings up another interesting point. Often, health providers have only seen brief videos online of subtle cataplexy and have not witnessed it in their office. If you have a video, this is an excellent opportunity to help educate your provider and clarify your diagnosis. After all, cataplexy cannot usually just be demonstrated on demand in the doctor's office. Indeed, the absence of sudden cataplexy after their attempts to prove cataplexy in their office would **not** rule this disorder out.

When patients deny having symptoms of cataplexy, I try to explain it and give them as many detailed descriptions as possible. I then ask them to go home and think about this symptom. I ask them to talk to their family and friends to see if they have noticed the patient having any unusual episodes. And remember, this symptom can develop over time and present several years after hypersomnia or excessive daytime sleepiness. So, I repeatedly ask them about cataplexy symptoms during subsequent visits, advise them to read and learn more about it, and recommend they talk to their families/friends.

I have my patients complete scales in my office, which we will review later, including an Epworth Sleepiness Scale and a Swiss Narcolepsy Scale. We also administer a Narcolepsy Assessment & Progress Screener (NAPS) scale and continue to increase their awareness of all the symptoms of Narcolepsy. The NAPS screener is a tool I recently helped to develop with my writing partners, Lewis J. Kass, M.D., and Laura B. Herpel, M.D. This screener evaluates the patient's perception of their sleepiness throughout the day, screens for specific cataplexy symptoms, screens for other medical, psychiatric, or other sleep disorders, and identifies the patient's particular goals for the future. We have also recently completed a pediatric/adolescent version of this scale. We will discuss these tools further in Chapter 4.

Presentations of Cataplexy

The list that follows describes some of the possible presentations of cataplexy.

- Head dropping and neck giving away
- Drooping eyelids
- Blurred vision
- Double vision
- Trouble focusing
- Raised eyebrows
- Slurred speech or garbled speech
- Stuttering
- Sagging jaw
- Tongue protrusion, unusual facial weakness, or movement
- Smile disruption
- Shoulder weakness
- Arm weakness
- Hand weakness and frequently dropping things (like cell phones)

- Inability to write/dropping pencil or pen
- Clumsiness or tripping over their feet
- Unexplained falls
- Leg or ankle weakness
- Knee buckling or knee unlocking
- Trembling of the knees from weakness alternating with contractions
- Complete collapse
- Feeling as if their body Is limp
- Slumping
- Melting
- Eyes fluttering
- Speech slurring or fading out
- Muscle jerks in the face or around the eyes
- Uneven smile
- Uneven opening of the eyes due to lid sagging
- "Almost stroke-like"
- Frequent or unexplained accidents, injuries, or wrecks. "I am accident-prone."

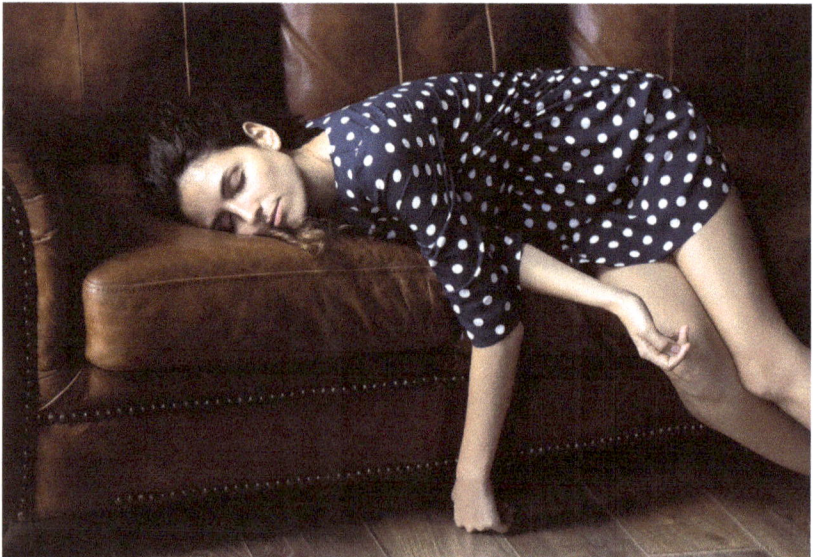

Remember, patients can move their eyes and continue to breathe during cataplexy (Schneider, L. and Elienbogen, 2020). They are aware of their surroundings. If the diagnosis is in question and their eyes are closed, raise their eyelids. Their eye response may help you determine that it is cataplexy. An excellent video of continued eye movement with facial cataplexy is in the Scheider and Ellenbogen article mentioned previously and referenced at the back of this book.

Patients may even avoid situations with strong emotional content to avoid cataplexy, resulting in further isolation. They may attempt to keep themselves emotionless, leading to increased concern from others about whether depression is present because the patient can look very flat and apathetic. It may have previously been misdiagnosed as a seizure, pseudo-seizures, hypoglycemia, POTS, a conversion disorder, fainting, a neuromuscular disorder, malingering, or "just faking it." Children with Narcolepsy can learn early to avoid birthday parties, trampolines, playgrounds, sleepovers, or other high-intensity situations to prevent cataplexy. I once had a patient whose facial expression was so entirely flat when I saw her that I was sure she had depression, and I asked her about it repeatedly for years. Later, she told me her kids had learned that if they got her really mad or laughing hard, they could get away with challenging behaviors because of her significant cataplexy, so she had trained herself to remain emotionless. Imagine that for a moment, growing up with an emotionless Mother!

Cataplexy can:

- Be vague.
- Occur in any muscle in the body (except for the eyes and the diaphragm).
- Occur with any emotion.
- Cause "Narcolepsy hands," in which the patient frequently drops things. (Be suspicious of those who say they often

have to replace their cell phones because they keep dropping them so much.)
- Be associated with rapid recovery after a few seconds or delayed even up to twenty minutes—when recovery occurs, it reverses quickly.
- Cause patients to learn suppression mechanisms to avoid increased emotions such as pain, anger, laughter, sexual excitation, fear, and humiliation to prevent cataplexy.
- Increase with poor sleep, fatigue, emotion, stress, or heavy meals.
- It can occur with loud noise or extremes of temperature.
- It can cause isolation and emotional distancing.

If cataplexy is present, it is helpful to identify the emotions associated with your cataplexy. Once identified, you can alert those around you of what emotions to be aware of. If laughter precipitates cataplexy, tell your family and friends not to tell jokes or make wisecracks while you are driving, going down the stairs, cooking, smoking, and hiking in unfamiliar territories. Narcolepsy patients need medical alert identification bracelets, badges, or necklaces. These can help people know how to respond. (We will discuss this more in Chapter 5.) It is important for everyone around the Narcoleptic patient having a cataplexy event to remain calm. The chaos, loud voices, anxiety over being the center of attention, and feeling flustered can all prolong the cataplexy event. Having a badge with instructions will calm those around you so they don't feel overwhelmed and upset thinking they must do something. (We have an offer for one of these badges at the back of the book.)

The sudden loss of muscle tone of cataplexy can be associated with the rapid return of muscle contraction. Recovery usually comes quickly and is complete. With the quick return of muscle function, it can almost look like a twitch, jerking, or a muscle "tic." (It is actually the reverse of a muscle "tic," defined as sudden muscle contraction and release.) It may look like a spasm. Some cataplexy events can be prolonged, or the patient may have consecutive short attacks. Occasionally, the patient can hallucinate during the cataplexy event, as this is a REM-associated phenomenon. Hypnogogic hallucinations are symptoms that may routinely be present with sleep, naps, and cataplexy.

Possible Triggers of Cataplexy

So, what are the possible triggers of cataplexy? It can be triggered by almost any strong emotional experience. Cataplexy can be a complete loss of muscle control or a partial loss of isolated muscle weakness. Overeem and associates (2011a) observed that approximately 60% of patients have spontaneous cataplexy, 15% have complete cataplexy lasting over two minutes, and 45% experience partial and complete cataplexy. Around a third of patients report only having partial cataplexy, with the jaw and the face more often involved in these partial attacks.

Treatment of cataplexy at this time includes medications such as oxybates, antidepressants, pitolisant, and even opioids (Heidbreder et al., 2020) have been reported to be helpful. Additional treatments are being considered. Behavioral and cognitive behavioral therapy are also used for cataplexy and will be discussed more in Chapter 5.

The following list provides some insight into possible cataplexy triggers, as noted in various studies and research:

- Stress
- Anger
- Happiness
- Being glad
- Exhilaration

- Fear
- Surprise
- Embarrassment
- Laughter
- Laughing excitedly
- Being tickled
- Feelings of joy (music, watching a movie, reading a book, watching a child graduate)
- Anticipation of saying something humorous
- Excitement
- Tension
- Sexual activity or arousal/excitement and orgasm
- Swimming
- Yawning
- Sadness
- Sorrow
- Being caught off guard
- Unexpectedly meeting a friend
- Annoyance
- Frustration
- Sighing
- Revulsion
- Severe Pain
- Humiliation
- Feeling flustered
- Being startled
- Feeling ashamed
- A loud noise
- Remembering a funny story
- Athletic endeavor

(Overeem et al., 2011b)(Quaedackers et al., 2021)(Krahn, L.E., Lymp, J.F., Moore, W.R., Slocumb N., 2005)

Cataplexy only occurs in Narcolepsy and can occur without a known trigger. So, when evaluating unusual symptoms such as cataplexy . . . Ask, ask, and ask them again!!! Ask everyone, even if they already have been diagnosed with Narcolepsy without cataplexy. Remember, this symptom can develop over time. It can change; therefore, your treatment plan must also change. It can change over time in severity; thus, alternative treatment interventions may become necessary. It can vary with stress levels. Always ask patients and their family members and friends about it.

Research on animals has led to many discoveries to advance Narcolepsy in the human population. Cataplexy can be seen in dogs, cats, and horses—especially Shetland ponies and Dobermans (Nishino, 2017). Cataplexy in dogs is usually triggered by emotionally rewarding behaviors such as eating, running, and social interaction and can cause postural collapse and weakness (Elliott & Swick, 2015).

One of my first exposures to cataplexy was watching *The Phil Donahue Show* years ago. He had a stage full of Narcoleptic dogs of various breeds that would all drop and have cataplexy when the audience clapped or laughed loudly. You can probably find this on YouTube and many other videos on cataplexy in people and pets. I saw one extreme video of a man in a tree with a power saw, and his friends were telling jokes below. This video was scary and unbelievable! There was another guy playing cards with his friends who would get him laughing, so he would have cataplexy in his hands and show them his cards. There are so many examples. I encourage you to look some up, such as "Dogs with Cataplexy," "Rusty the Narcoleptic Dog," "Narcoleptic Dogs with Emmanuel Mignot 2009," and "36-year-old horse during narcolepsy attack."

Unfortunately, I believe I saw this in my own home without realizing it in my Father, who had various medical/neurological issues and, unknown to us, a brain tumor. His head would fall so forward with the emotions/excitement of the holidays that his head would almost be in his plate of food. In our fear and anxiety about what we witnessed, we would very loudly try to "wake him up," which I now feel probably prolonged these episodes.

The assumption in the elderly with these symptoms is usually that they are over-prescribed or overtaking medications or that it is a progression of some other neurologic disease. It can just be cataplexy. An interesting video of facial cataplexy demonstrating persistent eye movements in an elderly patient can be found in a link provided in an article by Schneider and Ellenbogen (2020) referenced at the back of the book.

Cataplexy can occur in children and adolescents; we will discuss this in detail in Chapter 6. Normal infants and small children have increased REM sleep early in their development. There are many videos of infants demonstrating REM-related atonia that is normal for their age. These videos provide some realistic examples of what abnormal REM-related phenomena may look like later in life in those with Narcolepsy. Keep that in mind when you see children falling asleep in unusual situations or suddenly losing muscle control when falling asleep. Some children with Narcolepsy have static cataplexy and unique presentations (Serra et al., 2008a) and "cataplectic facies" without emotion (Anic-Labat et al., 1999a). I would suggest you look up these references and check them out.

So, remember, cataplexy is usually brief, transient, may present in various ways, follows an emotional trigger, may be recognized first by others, spontaneously recovers, may be subtle, may be very dramatic, and at times can even be dangerous if it occurs while walking down stairs, driving, or walking across the street. Now, let's move on to the symptoms of disrupted nocturnal sleep and insomnia with Narcolepsy.

Chapter 3

"You Can't Have Insomnia if You Have Narcolepsy!?!"

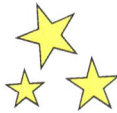

Disrupted Nocturnal Sleep in the Narcolepsy Patient

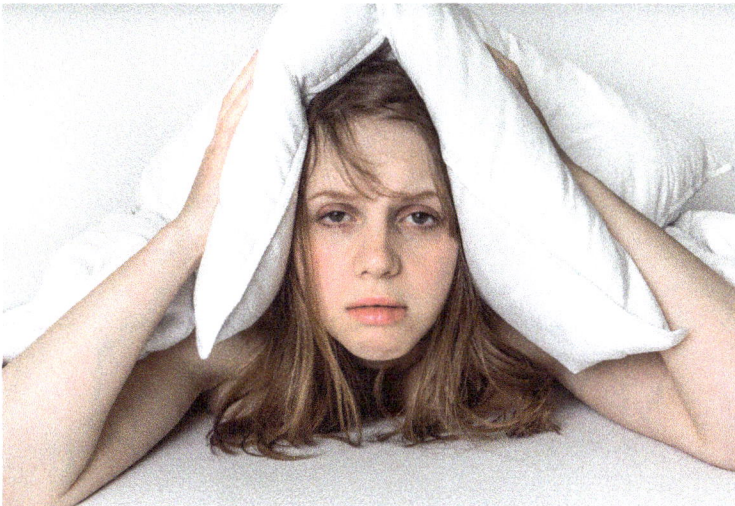

"When you have insomnia, you're never really asleep,
and you're never really awake."
From the movie Fight Club, based on the novel by Chuck Palahniuk

Did you know that although people with Narcolepsy are very sleepy, they do not sleep well? They have sleep-wake instability. No matter how long an unmedicated Narcolepsy patient sleeps, their brain sleeps incorrectly. They can fall asleep quickly, but their sleep is light and fragmented. They have frequent arousals. They sleep in the lighter stages of sleep. Their REM sleep may occur soon after sleep onset. They may have disruptions of REM sleep and other disorders such as REM Sleep Behavior Disorder (RBD). They have very vivid dreams and sometimes severe nightmares. It may be difficult for them to distinguish between dreaming and reality, and they can become almost delusional in the belief that something truly happened that they just dreamed about. Unfortunately, these sleep issues can lead to anticipatory insomnia, nighttime sleep avoidance, and skipping of the recommended daytime naps.

Many of the associated symptoms or other disorders related to Narcolepsy can also be disruptive to sleep, such as hypnogogic hallucinations, sleep paralysis, rapid eye movement sleep behavior disorder, nightmares, restless legs syndrome, periodic limb movement disorder, nocturnal eating, sleep apnea, depression, and anxiety (Maski et al., 2022).

I say this repeatedly in this book, but I think it is essential to define the point clearly: **Narcolepsy is a 24-hour-a-day disorder!** We need to stabilize both sleep and wake in the treatment of Narcolepsy. I once had a patient tell me that her sleep doctor told her she could not possibly have Narcolepsy if she had insomnia. This is not true! Insomnia can cause significant distress. Disruptions due to both hypersomnia and insomnia create great chaos in the Narcolepsy patient's life.

Sometimes, there is a "blaming" quality to the recommendations from family members, friends, and providers about controlling these symptoms, further contributing to the shame often felt in patients with Narcolepsy. Statements made in an attempt to be helpful include things like: "If only you would not nap during the day, you would sleep better at night," "You sleep all the time. How could you have insomnia?" "You just need to turn things off and sleep better at night, and you would do better during the day," "You just need to stop all caffeine," or even "You just need to drink more caffeine during the day . . . have you tried Red Bull?" In an attempt to help, they may frustrate the situation. Often, others want to help so much and are frustrated and feel powerless. So, after reading, please share this book and your insights with others to give them some tools to help you. Let's educate and show them how they can be more helpful!

"At night, I can't sleep. In the morning, I can't wake up."

Unknown

Decreased amounts of slow-wave sleep indicate Narcoleptics do not get the deeper, more restorative sleep of stage 3 NREM sleep, which is especially physically beneficial. In the morning, they frequently have "sleep inertia," which is temporary disorientation, inability to wake up fully, and decline in performance (slower reaction time, decreased short-term memory, reduced ability to remember things, and slower learning speed). This piece of the puzzle is often missed by others who think, "You sleep all the time; how could you be sleepy?" This often leads to frustration on both sides and even more isolation for the person with Narcolepsy, demonstrating why such a comprehensive treatment plan is required to address all symptoms and areas of disabilities.

"Prioritizing good sleep is good self-love."

Danielle Laporte

Nightmares are also an issue for some Narcoleptic patients. The nightmares can be so severe that patients are afraid to sleep, worsening sleep deprivation and excessive daytime sleepiness. Patients may be so fearful of hypnogogic hallucinations and nightmares that they will not take the suggested scheduled daytime naps either. There are medications for nightmares, such as Prazosin (Minipress), some antidepressants, and cognitive behavioral therapy (CBT) and imagery rehearsal therapy (IRT), which we will discuss later. Detailed treatment recommendations for insomnia are discussed in greater detail in Chapter 5.

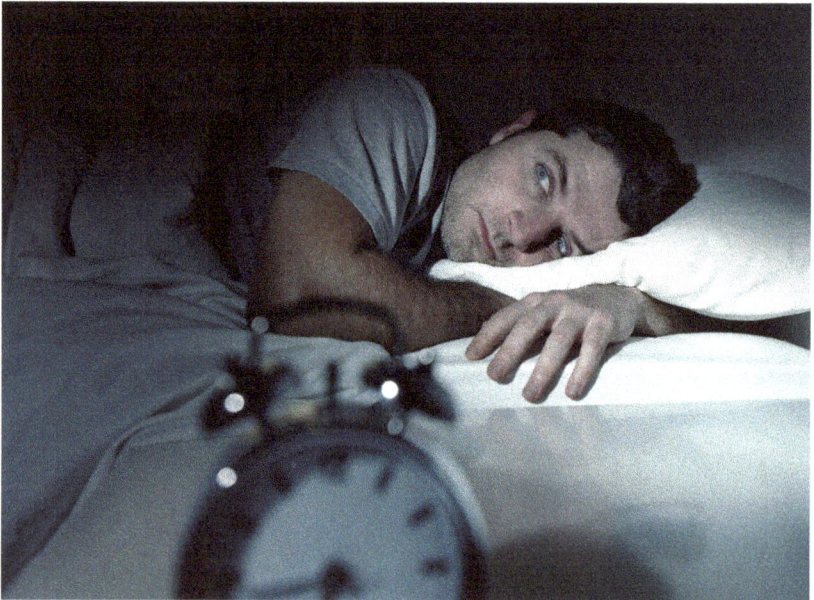

*"Dear Sleep, I'm sorry we broke up this morning.
I'll do anything to get you back!"*

Anonymous

Chapter 4

"Answers, Please!"

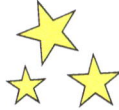

Diagnosing Narcolepsy

"It's like somebody gave me a puzzle, but I don't have the box with the picture on it. So, I don't know what the final thing is supposed to look like. I'm not even sure I have all the pieces . . ."

Sharon Draper in "Out of My Mind"

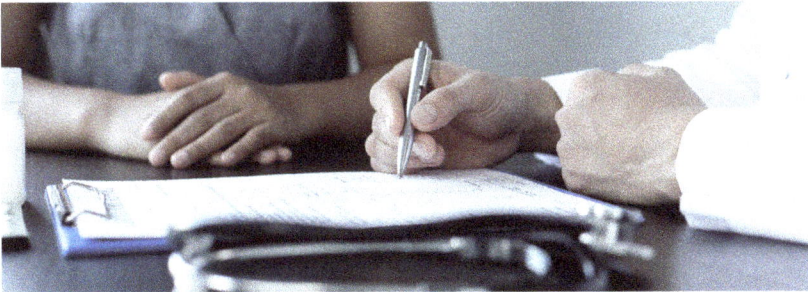

"Because doctors can't name the illness, everyone—the patient's family, friends, health insurance, and in many cases the patient—comes to think of the patient as not really sick and not really suffering. What the patient comes to require in these circumstances, in the absence of help, are facts—tests, and studies that show that they might 'in fact' have something."

Joseph Dumit

The journey to diagnosing Narcolepsy can be long and turbulent because it's often not just Narcolepsy impacting the patient—in many cases, there are associations with other sleep disorders and health issues like depression, anxiety, and chronic pain. These can cloud the picture and prevent the patient, providers, and family from seeing the sleep disorder right before their eyes. As a starting point, evaluating the items below will be highly beneficial to light the way:

- A detailed sleep history and investigation into unusual sleep symptoms or behaviors
- A review of any medications, over-the-counter medications, or supplements
- Daytime and nighttime schedules
- Associated symptoms of other disorders (sleep disorders, poor sleep hygiene, depression, anxiety, substance use, and other observations)

The various evaluations and examinations that follow are some potential next steps the patient can take to investigate their symptoms and gain a diagnosis.

Detailed Sleep History: The sleep history should include things such as: How long have you had the issue? What makes it better or worse? Are there any associated psychiatric or medical problems? What have you tried already? How is your sleeping environment? Is your mattress comfortable? Does your partner snore? Do you have children in the bed? Are there pets in the bed? How is the temperature in the room? Is your room noisy (trains, cars, busy streets), or is your room dark enough? What is your bedtime routine? Do you read/ watch tv/ hang out in bed? Are you taking any medications at night? Are you taking any sleep aids? Is your sleep schedule consistent? Do you nap during the day or in the evening? Do you have other sleep disorder symptoms? Do you drink alcohol? Do you have reflux or heartburn? Do you have to get up at night to go to the bathroom? Is chronic pain contributing to your sleep disruption?

Cataplexy Diary: This diary is used to mark the frequency and specific symptoms of cataplexy. One should describe in as much detail as possible the presentation of each cataplexy episode as they may change over time. Have others help you with this. Describe the emotion or situation that precipitated the cataplexy. Report what muscles were involved. Estimate how long it occurred. Consider what things or situations may have contributed.

Sleep Diary: A sleep diary includes things like when you went to sleep, when you got up, how many awakenings you felt you had, what woke you up, did you have caffeine late in the day, did you drink alcohol, did you nap, and did you take medications. This should be kept two weeks before your sleep study.

Polysomnography (PSG) (Spriggs, 2014): The PSG (or overnight sleep study) involves brain EEG leads placed superficially on the head to monitor sleep staging and eye leads to measure eye movements to help with sleep staging and to document the onset of REM sleep, along with EMG evaluation to evaluate the absence of movements during REM sleep, bruxism (teeth grinding), leg movements, and abnormal movements during REM sleep. The PSG is used to evaluate for sleep disorders such as snoring, obstructive sleep apnea, central sleep apnea, restless legs syndrome, periodic limb movement disorder, sleep fragmentation, the presence or absence of slow wave sleep, REM sleep behavior disorder, sleep talking, sleep-wake misperception, and (with additional EEG leads) it can also help in the diagnosis of epilepsy. The assessment includes airflow, respiratory effort, an EKG to evaluate for arrhythmias, and sound recordings to measure snoring. Video monitoring will also be obtained. The PSG examination is also necessary before a Multiple Sleep Latency Test (MSLT) to aid in diagnosing Narcolepsy.

Multiple Sleep Latency Test (MSLT) (Carskadon, 1986b): The MSLT examination (or daytime nap study) is used to diagnose Narcolepsy and Idiopathic Hypersomnia. It always follows a PSG examination, and the patient is given up to five naps to sleep, each two hours apart. The patient is given twenty minutes to fall asleep, and during the test, the presence or absence of REM sleep is documented, along with a measure of the average time to fall asleep. For the diagnosis of Narcolepsy to be confirmed, the patient must have at least two sleep onset REM periods (a sleep onset REM period on the overnight PSG can also count towards this number), and the mean sleep onset latency must be low (less than eight minutes).

False negatives can occur on the MSLT due to certain medications, environmental noise, anxiety, performance anxiety, etc. Examples of drugs interfering with test results would be decreased REM sleep with antidepressants and benzodiazepines (such as Xanax, Ativan, Valium, or Klonopin). A more complete list of medications that interfere with the MSLT is discussed by Krahn, Arand, Avidan, et al. (Krahn et al., 2021). It is essential to consider these things in interpreting the data from the MSLT. If the medicines are not reviewed adequately, an MSLT test may falsely be reported as negative.

Also, chronic sleep deprivation and shift work can influence the results of the MSLT. In order to get accurate results, every attempt should be made to normalize your sleep at least two weeks before the MSLT. Marijuana use can also influence the outcome.

Another sleep disorder evaluated by the MSLT findings and discussed previously includes Idiopathic Hypersomnia (IH). Patients with Idiopathic Hypersomnia fall asleep quickly but do not meet the REM criteria for diagnosing Narcolepsy and do not have cataplexy. To diagnose Idiopathic Hypersomnia, the patient will have a decreased sleep onset latency of less than or equal to eight minutes and a history of sleeping up to twelve to fourteen hours daily. The MSLT and patient history of whether cataplexy is present are used to rule out Narcolepsy before IH can be diagnosed. Patients with Idiopathic Hypersomnia also complain of sleep inertia, which is extreme difficulty waking up in the morning, and this can be seen in Narcolepsy.

Additionally, other causes of sleep disruption must also be eliminated.

Epworth Sleepiness Scale (ESS) (Johns, 1991): This questionnaire evaluates a patient's degree of sleepiness in various situations such as sitting and reading, watching TV, sitting inactive in a public place, as a passenger in a car, lying down to rest, sitting and talking, sitting quietly after a meal without alcohol, and in a car while stopped for a few minutes. There is also a child and adolescent form (ESS-CHAD Wang et al., 2017).

Stanford Sleepiness Scale (SSS) (Hoddes et al., 1973): This test measures sleepiness on a scale of 1–7. It is based on sleepiness descriptions such as feeling active, vital, alert, and wide awake; functioning at a high level, but not peak; relaxed, awake, but not fully alert; foggy, not at peak, let down; sleepy, fighting sleep, prefer to be laying down; almost asleep, sleep onset coming soon and losing the ability to stay awake.

Swiss Narcolepsy Scale (SNS) (Sturzenegger, C. et al., 2014): This form includes five questions rated on a scale of 1–5, including: How often are you unable to fall asleep? How often do you feel bad or not well-rested in the morning? How often do you take a nap during the day? How often have you experienced weak knees/ bucking of the knees during emotions like laughing, happiness, or anger? And how often have you experienced sagging of the jaw during emotions like laughing, happiness, or anger? A formula calculates a total score on this test to indicate the presence of Narcolepsy with cataplexy.

Karolinska Sleepiness Scale (Shahid et al., 2011): This scale measures the subjective level of situational sleepiness at a particular time of the day over the last ten minutes and includes the following: Extremely alert; very alert; alert; rather alert; neither alert nor sleepy; some signs of sleepiness; sleepy but no effort to keep awake; sleepy but some effort to stay awake; very sleepy, significant effort to keep awake, fighting sleep; and finally extremely sleepy, can't stay awake.

Ullanlinna Narcolepsy Scale (Hublin et al., 1994): This test is an 11-item scale to evaluate Narcolepsy symptoms and their frequency, including questions such as: how fast do you usually fall asleep in the evening, do you sleep during the day, do you fall asleep unintentionally during the day, and if so how likely is it in the following situations: reading, traveling, standing, eating, or other unusual conditions. This scale also asks the patient if, while laughing, glad, angry, or in other exciting situations, they have episodes of knees unlocking, mouth opening, head nodding, or falling, and if so, how often.

Narcolepsy Assessment & Progress Screener (NAPS) (Stultz, Herpel, & Kass 2023): This is a new sleep screener created by Laura B. Herpel, M.D., Lewis Kass, M.D., and myself, which has a patient version and a family/friend version to obtain information on the overall rating of sleepiness, sleepiness severity at different times during the day, to what extent the sleepiness results in avoiding social interactions, to what capacity sleepiness affects work/school, specific activities where sleepiness impairs their ability to function, how many times a day the patient naps, symptoms of cataplexy, vivid dreams/nightmares, sleep paralysis, hypnogogic hallucinations, disrupted nocturnal sleep/awakenings, the presence of other sleep disorder symptoms, contributing factors, things that could disrupt sleep, and goals for treatment.

The Friends and Family version of the NAPS screener includes questions such as:

- Have you noticed that your family member or friend experiences excessive daytime sleepiness? Do they seem to nap more frequently than others?
- Have you noticed them having unusual muscle weakness with emotions?
- Have you noticed other family members with excessive daytime sleepiness?
- Can you describe areas within your friend's or family member's life where they may be affected by extreme daytime sleepiness?

This scale allows the patient and their friend/family member to have areas of open descriptions of issues in their own words. It lists goals to monitor for the future and areas of impairment to follow. I have included a copy of this screener in Appendix #1.

Pediatric Narcolepsy Assessment & Progress Screener (PED-NAPS) (Stultz, Kass, & Herpel 2023): This assessment includes questions on excessive sleepiness, hyperactivity, increased sleep, school issues, sudden weight gain, pediatric presentations of cataplexy, listing three ways their sleep issues have impaired their ability to function, and three goals for the future. A copy of this scale is also available in Appendix #2.

The Cataplexy Emotional Trigger Questionnaire (Moore et al., 2007): This screener includes questions about sudden muscle weakness and associated symptoms of cataplexy. Questions include: Have you EVER experienced sudden muscle weakness when you laugh? Can you hear? Does your speech ever become slurred? Is your head affected? Is your whole body affected?

Visual Analog Scale-Sleep Inertia (VAS-SI) (Dauvilliers et al., 2023)**:** This test evaluates the patient's difficulty getting up in the morning. It is a self-reported scale between 0 to 100 in which patients grade the question, "How difficult was it for you to wake up this morning? A score closer to 100 indicates it is very difficult." It is used to evaluate sleep inertia or "sleep drunkenness."

The Maintenance of Wakefulness Test (MWT) (Mitler et al., 1982): This test is almost the reverse of an MSLT examination in which the patient is given four 40-minute nap opportunities in the sleep lab in a quiet, dimly lit room and asked to stay awake. The test is repeated at two-hour intervals. A value of less than eight minutes is considered abnormal.

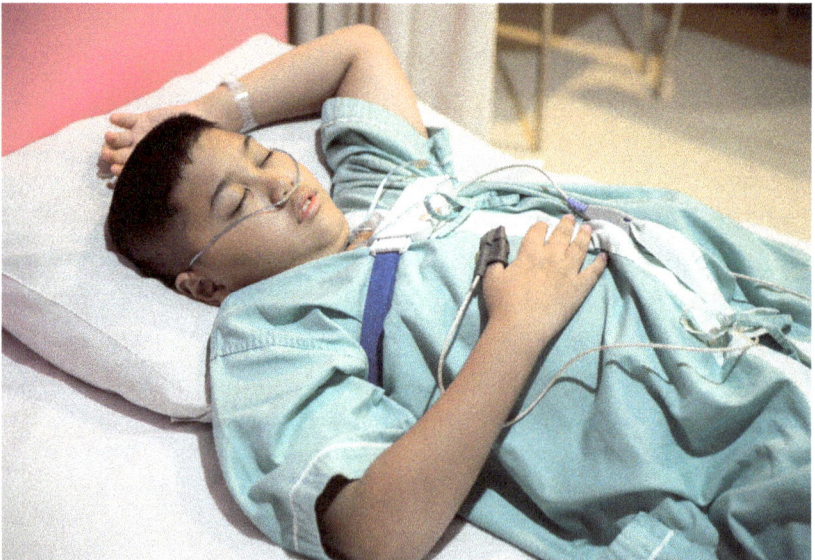

"Being at ease with not knowing is crucial for answers to come to you."

Eckhart Tolle

The author John Gray is quoted as saying, "When the student is ready, the teacher appears. When the question is asked then, the answer is heard. When we are truly ready to receive, then what we need will become available." I like this quote, and I believe it is true. However, with Narcolepsy, sometimes the journey is much more complicated. If you suspect you or a family member may have Narcolepsy and have had difficulty getting to the diagnosis, find a doctor familiar with sleep disorders other than just sleep apnea. Some sleep physicians focus primarily on treating sleep apnea and managing CPAP and may rarely focus on treating insomnia or identifying other causes of hypersomnia. For those with significant apnea and respiratory issues, that is undoubtedly necessary. But if hypersomnia continues or sleep apnea has been ruled out, we should look at other possible sleep disorders and contributing factors.

If the MSLT is negative, then further evaluation and consideration are necessary. It is never just one, and you are done if you have a negative MSLT. One negative MSLT examination does not exclude the diagnosis of Narcolepsy. There may be contributing factors such as what medicines the patient is on during the study, how long the patient stopped meds before the study, anxiety, noise, and comfort. All of these things can be disruptive to the normal sleep process. Anything that disrupts a patient's regular sleep could impair the results. Repeating the study may be necessary if the MSLT is negative, but the symptoms are still suspicious. We would not do one EKG to rule out a heart attack in a patient with chest pain and stop there. We would continue to evaluate, and they would have repeat EKG examinations if symptoms persist. The same is true with Narcolepsy and continued hypersomnia.

Suppose a patient has excessive sleepiness and cataplexy. In that case, they can also get the diagnosis of Narcolepsy with cataplexy using the DSM-V criteria, even if the MSLT is negative or not completed. (Where possible, it is better to get the positive MSLT to aid in insurance coverage and, if necessary, future disability issues.) The DSM-V criteria include excessive daytime sleepiness at least three times per week over three months with **any** of the following: cataplexy occurring at least a few times per month, decreased cerebrospinal fluid hypocretin levels, or an abnormal PSG/MSLT.

Medications that may interfere with sleep architecture and the PSG/MSLT results (Krahn et al., 2021) can include things like donepezil, theophylline, caffeine, gabapentin, SSRI antidepressants, SNRI antidepressants, bupropion, tricyclic antidepressants, Benadryl and other sedating antihistamines, antipsychotics, antihypertensives, benzodiazepines (such as Xanax, Klonopin, Ativan, Valium), Lithium, meds used for restless legs syndrome such as Requip or Mirapex, sleeping pills such as ramelteon, Hetlioz (tasimelteon), pain meds such as Methadone, hydrocodone, suvorexant, any of the sodium oxybates or their derivatives (Xyrem, Xywav, or Lumryz), steroids such as prednisone, wake-promoting agents such as armodafinil, modafinil, pitolisant, solriameftol, and one that is often overlooked is marijuana.

In an ideal world, we stop any medications we fear may interfere with the test before the study based on how long the substance stays in the system. That is not always possible. Before interpreting the results, the medicines taken around the time and during the MSLT study should be listed on the actual MSLT report to reveal the most conclusive results. For example, sometimes depression and anxiety are so significant that we cannot stop the antidepressants before the study. These medications can effect the outcome of the study. If a patient is on an antidepressant, I will dictate that in my report.

When you know you are going to have a sleep study, stop stimulants and wake-promoting meds one to two weeks before the study, antidepressants three to four weeks before the study, and discontinue marijuana use at least three weeks or more before the study as well. If you cannot stop the medicine or THC, try keeping the use levels steady so they may be considered when interpreting the study results. Let the provider know what and how much you are taking.

If the answers are not clear, always keep looking! If you still have symptoms, you may need to repeat the study.

If your tests are negative, the diagnosis may be Idiopathic Hypersomnia with prolonged nighttime and daytime sleep, continued excessive daytime sleepiness, the absence of cataplexy, great difficulty waking up associated with "sleep drunkenness," memory issues, and automatic behavior. The recent FDA approval of Xywav for this Disorder and the recent FDA approval of Wakix (pitilosant) as Orphan Drug designation for IH treatment has helped bring this disorder to light. For those who may be diagnosed with Idiopathic Hypersomnia instead of Narcolepsy, I would strongly suggest you visit the Hypersomnia Foundation on the internet at www.hypersomniafoundation.org.

As stated previously, there are other associated disorders (sleep, medical, and psychiatric) with an increased prevalence occurring with Narcolepsy. Sometimes, these co-occurring disorders can complicate the clinical presentation of Narcolepsy. These disorders can co-exist, and the presence of one does not exclude the diagnosis of Narcolepsy. I believe these conditions will need to be treated simultaneously. You would not wait to treat the Narcolepsy symptoms until after you treat all the depression and anxiety, any more than waiting to treat diabetes until your blood pressure is controlled if both disorders were present. Your treatment options may vary based on your co-existing conditions. We will discuss this more in Chapter 5. Just know sleep disorders run hand in hand with many other diseases. A chronic sleep disorder such as Narcolepsy, with its multiple hardships and failures before the actual diagnosis, can lead to depression and anxiety, and the sleep disruption of Narcolepsy can contribute to various physical and mental health issues. Depression, anxiety, and Narcolepsy are discussed in greater detail in Chapter 7.

"I'm trying to find answers. It can be quite frustrating, but at the same time, I'm never quite satisfied with what I'm doing, so I'm always looking for the next thing."

Robert Longo

Chapter 5

"Let's Talk About Treatment!"

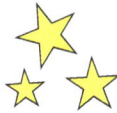

⭐⭐⭐

Medication and Behavioral Treatments of Narcolepsy

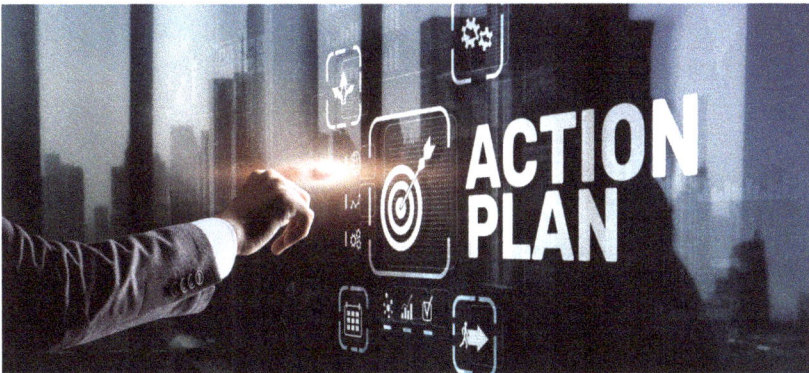

"Happiness is a nice long nap."
Peanuts

How many unusable hours do you have during the day? Treatment of this disorder involves medication, education, committed behavioral therapy, and a multifocal treatment plan involving educating those around you and making appropriate accommodations academically or occupationally. You need to look for resources and never stop looking. Your illness will change over time, treatment options will change over time, and your available resources will change over time. Narcolepsy is a journey, a marathon . . . not a sprint. There will be lots of trial and error.

You may benefit from cognitive behavioral therapy for your hypersomnia/excessive daytime sleepiness (Ong et al., 2020), cognitive behavioral therapy for cataplexy (Marín Agudelo et al., 2014), and the cognitive behavioral treatment of insomnia (Morin et al., 2009) (Mitchell et al., 2012). Cognitive restructuring, breathing exercises, progressive muscle relaxation, stimulus control, meditation, hypnosis, biofeedback, sleep environment changes, lifestyle changes, limiting time in bed, using the bed for sleep and sex only, increased exercise, a hot bath or shower one hour before bedtime, a "mental wind down" limiting stimulation one to two hours before bed, decreased caffeine, light muscle stretching, and limiting alcohol or excessive fluids for a couple of hours before bedtime can all be helpful techniques to aid in treating insomnia associated with your disorder. Digital cognitive behavioral therapy for insomnia has been studied to be beneficial, especially when used with medication therapy (Lu et al., 2023). Cognitive behavioral therapy can also be helpful for any co-existing depression and anxiety.

Knowledge Is Power!

The first step in treatment is learning all you possibly can about Narcolepsy and what may be your specific triggers to cataplexy. You will also need to help educate your family and those around you. If laughter is your trigger for cataplexy, they should be instructed not to tell jokes when you are in situations that may be dangerous should you fall or lose muscle control. Helping them understand the need for naps and structured sleep is also essential to the treatment plan. We will talk more about education for the family in Chapter 9.

There are degrees of Narcolepsy, not unlike other disorders such as diabetes. There are diabetics on multiple medications and high doses of insulin, and some that take just one pill to control their disease. Other patients can mostly control their blood sugar with diet, exercise, and behavioral interventions. The same is true for Narcolepsy; however, medications are an essential part of the treatment plan in most patients. Sleep hygiene and scheduled naps are always a part of our behavioral treatment plan. I can so clearly remember my sleep colleague and friend Dr. Richard Bogan giving a lecture on the treatment of Narcolepsy, stating, "There is a nap for that!" I can't emphasize enough how important napping is in treating Narcolepsy!

"Naptime is my Happy Hour."

Anonymous

Narcolepsy patients fight being sleepy so much it almost feels like a failure to give up and take a nap during the day, but they are often so necessary. I use a cell phone metaphor to explain the importance of a nap to my patients. If your cell phone starts to die during the day, you at some point have to stop, plug it in, and give it time to recharge, or the battery dies out, and the phone becomes useless to you. Naps are used to recharge. Sometimes, we have to figure out what nap length is too much or too little for the patient with Narcolepsy. We recommend one or two scheduled naps of around 15–30 minutes long, depending on your day and evening responsibilities and the severity of your Narcolepsy. Naps are needed to recharge when you have periods of extreme sleepiness. So, we must consider what time of the day patients are most sleepy to determine the nap's timing and length. Dr. Harpel, Dr. Kass, and I think the NAPS screener we developed helps determine the timing of naps and additional medication adjustments (see Appendix 1 and 2) necessary and is a benefit of that specific screener.

Additionally, we must continue to look at contributing factors, even in patients with known Narcolepsy. I have one patient with significant Narcolepsy who is on various medications and keeps asking for more, but she only sleeps five to six hours per night and does not nap because of her job demands. Sleep deprivation is clearly a contributing factor in this case. We can rarely get ahead of the excessive daytime sleepiness of Narcolepsy if the patient is consistently sleep-deprived and not allowing enough time for rest. Meds can't fix that, even in those without Narcolepsy.

One of the first things I must emphasize is the need for you to discuss your symptoms (and **all** of your symptoms—even those related to sex) with your provider! A study of 200 patients and 251 physicians called the "Burden of Narcolepsy: A Survey of Patients and Physicians" (Thorpy et al., 2019) revealed that 39% of patients were not discussing with their providers the negative impacts of their Narcolepsy on work/school performance, interpersonal relationships, and social activities. And 50% did not discuss how it affects them emotionally. Additionally, physicians reported that the patient's Narcolepsy symptoms were entirely or primarily controlled in 27.5% of patients, but only 12% of the patients felt their symptoms were adequately controlled. We all need to work better as a team.

I heard a lecture once that said the goal of our treatment in Narcolepsy should be "Wakefulness, not just a lack of sleepiness." The quote stayed with me, but I cannot remember who said it. This comment really struck home for me. We have to be aggressive about identifying patient-specific treatment goals. On the NAPS screener that I mentioned previously, the patient lists their top three treatment goals. The end goal is not just an improvement on the Epworth Sleepiness Scale! We must look at what the patient needs specifically. And we have to look at morning, afternoon, and evening symptoms to provide treatments when most needed. In the screener, we have them rate their sleepiness on a scale of 0–10, with ten being the most severe from 8:00 a.m. to noon, noon to 6:00 p.m., and 6:00 p.m. to 10:00 p.m. so that we can customize their treatment based on their requirements during those periods.

The Use of Medications

Before I go on, let me clarify that I use all these medications and am not endorsing one over the other. This book does not comprehensively review medications, side effects, and risks. I refer you to your provider for a complete review of treatment options. General discussions are provided to give an overall picture of the current pharmacological interventions possible. However, I like the medicines that are approved to treat both the excessive daytime sleepiness and cataplexy at the same time, such as Xyrem (sodium oxybate), Xywav (calcium, magnesium, potassium, sodium oxybate), Lumryz (the long-acting sodium oxybate), and Wakix (pitolisant) because these meds may allow you to prescribe a fewer number of medications in some patients that have both sleepiness and cataplexy. Wakix (pitolisant) is the only non-controlled medication in this group and is a beneficial intervention.

One of the oxybates may be more advantageous for those with significant sleep disruption. However, if there is frequent alcohol use, oxybate medications must be avoided, as you cannot take them with alcohol. If alcohol is used only occasionally (like during the holidays), patients can still be prescribed an oxybate medicine but would need to **hold it and not take it on any night they use**

alcohol. If there are blood pressure or cardiac issues, stimulants, Wakix (pitolisant), and some antidepressants may need to be avoided or decreased in dosage. Sunosi (solriameftol) can increase blood pressure and needs to be considered before starting in those whose blood pressure is uncontrolled. Monitoring blood pressure after starting is essential with Sunosi (solriamfetol) and the stimulants. Decreased appetite and possibly reduced weight can be found in those using stimulants.

But all these medicines have their place. Most frequently, in Narcolepsy, we use a layering of meds and must use a combination. We often have to add a sprinkle of a short-acting stimulant medicine in the late afternoon as a PRN medication to ensure patients remain productive and present for their family and other social commitments after work or school. Once again, using the metaphor of diabetes, we would not just treat the daytime symptoms of diabetes and ignore their nighttime or evening issues. After all, Narcolepsy is a 24-hour illness!

We also know that patients go through spells that, for whatever reason, a treatment plan that was successful for an extended period will suddenly need a change up or an additional medication. We must always consider whether we are actually "as good as it gets" and sometimes adjust up and then back off if not needed or give a PRN and monitor how often we must use it. We are fortunate in the field of Narcolepsy, as there has been an explosion of new medications and ideas for others in the last few years. Knowledge about this disorder and possible treatment interventions are expanding very rapidly. Any comments I make on medicines will likely need to be updated as soon as the book is published. Still, I am including a general summary to familiarize you with at least the names of the current medications available. Continue to check with your provider and look for updates on available treatments at Wake Up Narcolepsy, Project Sleep, The Narcolepsy Network, and other reliable resources.

"Treatment originates outside you; healing comes from within."

Andrew Weil

And, in the words of Deborah Tannen, "Treating people the same is not equal treatment if they are not the same." I very much agree with this statement. Everyone needs an individualized treatment plan tailored to their schedules and work/family demands. There is no one-size-fits-all approach! Elderly patients may have multiple co-existing disorders and be on various medications, requiring dosing modifications of meds and even different behavioral changes. Younger children often have a higher metabolism and fewer co-existing things to consider but are smaller. Hormonal changes in adolescents may change the degree of sleepiness and require medication adjustments, especially around the menstrual cycle. Pregnant women need frank discussions about medications and whether to use them during pregnancy. Other safety and behavioral recommendations must be followed aggressively when patients with Narcolepsy do not use meds during their pregnancy. They may need PRN medications when their excessive daytime sleepiness becomes almost dangerous to them and their unborn child. After delivery, issues also arise if they are breastfeeding. If job schedules change, work demands change, and family issues arise, then temporary medication demands may also vary. Menopausal and perimenopausal periods may require increased dosing of medications. Treatment of this disorder must be a fluid process.

"The question is not how to get cured, but how to live."

Joseph Conrad

An Overview of Narcolepsy Medications

Now, let's review some medications used to treat Narcolepsy. Remember to always look for new options. I am only listing meds that have been tried at the time of writing to familiarize you with medication names. And once again, by the time this book is published, there will probably be new options, and this list may be outdated. A list of medications potentially used, including both generic and brand names, is included at the back of this book to help you become familiar with the medicines potentially prescribed.

The Oxybates: Xyrem/Xywav/Lumryz: Sodium oxybate was one of the first unique and more specific medications for Narcolepsy and has been a game changer for this disorder! Xyrem (sodium oxybate) and its next-generation Xywav (calcium, magnesium, potassium, and sodium oxybate) may be a building block to the foundation of our often layered treatments of Narcolepsy. These medications are taken at night and are repeated once during the night. A recently released once-nightly form called Lumryz may benefit some, especially those who do not wake up in time to remember their second dose. Xywav is the second generation of Xyrem with decreased sodium, which provides a protective benefit, especially given the possibility of increased cardiovascular issues associated with Narcolepsy, as reported in the "Burden of Narcolepsy Disease" study (Black et al., 2017).

Once-nightly dosing has been used more frequently with Xywav in treating Idiopathic Hypersomnia, but two doses are currently recommended for treating Narcolepsy. I am convinced that one of these medications' many benefits is the sleep schedule it causes patients to maintain. Detailed instructions are given to patients on how to use this medication, such as avoiding food two hours before dosing, getting their pajamas on and in bed before taking the drug, and not using it with alcohol. I believe this helps patients pay attention to their sleep and their schedule. The oxybates, we believe, work on GABA in the brain. These medications are tapered up and must build up in the system for full effectiveness. Xyrem and Xywav can be used in children from seven years of age. Maski and associates reported that intrinsic sleep instability with Narcolepsy improves with sodium oxybate, but the risks and benefits should be discussed with patients (2022).

Wake-Promoting Agents and Stimulants: Somnolytics, which aid in decreasing daytime sedation, include Wakix (pitolisant), Provigil (modafinil), Nuvigil (armodafinil), Sunosi (solriamfetol,) and the psychostimulants such as Ritalin or Concerta (methylphenidate), Adderall (dextroamphetamine/amphetamine), Vyvanse (lisdexamfetamine), Focalin (dexmethylphenidate), Zenzedi (dextroamphetamine sulfate), or Dexedrine (dextroamphetamine). Provigil (modafinil) and Nuvigil (armodafinil) work on dopamine and noradrenergic areas. Modafinil has been used since the 1980s in the treatment of Narcolepsy. A newer formulation is being investigated of modafinil with flecainide (Thorpy, 2020).

 Stimulant medications provide some advantages in offering both long-acting and short-acting versions, which may be combined to control symptoms throughout the day. The short-acting stimulants are often used as PRN medications in combination with the various other medications used to treat Narcolepsy as well, for symptoms that occur later in the day, when having to drive for extended periods, during more stressful times, when there is co-existing ADHD, if "brain fog" is present, and when hormonal changes intermittently appear and are contributing to hypersomnia, to name a few situations.

Thomas Scammell, MD, in his *UpToDate* article entitled "Treatment of Narcolepsy in adults" (Scammell, 2023), provided an excellent diagram for the symptomatic management of Narcolepsy in adults. He suggested we first look at things that could worsen sleepiness, such as medications with sedating side effects like benzodiazepines, opioids, antipsychotics, and alcohol. As well as looking at things contributing to insomnia, such as excessive caffeine use or theophylline. In addition to behavioral recommendations, he then suggested modafinil/armodafinil (preferred), pitolisant, and solriamfetol are the first-line wake-promoting meds, with pitolisant being preferred if co-existing cataplexy is present. Adding a second wake-promoting drug or stimulant may be helpful if symptoms continue. With ongoing sleepiness or cataplexy, oxybates should be considered. For ongoing cataplexy, venlafaxine, fluoxetine, duloxetine, tricyclic antidepressants, pitolisant, or oxybates are treatment options.

Wakix (pitolisant): Now, let's talk about pitolisant in more detail. Wakix (pitolisant) has a unique action and increases the synthesis and release of histamine. It is FDA-approved for treating both the excessive daytime sleepiness and cataplexy of Narcolepsy and is a non-controlled treatment for Narcolepsy. It can be provided with refills, contributing to its ease of use. Pitolisant takes time to build up in the system (like oxybates and antidepressants). We also start with a lower dose and taper up to a higher dose based on what other medications the patient is taking. It takes patience to allow this medication to build up and reach its maximum effectiveness. Still, with time, it can be an extremely beneficial medication in Narcolepsy or Idiopathic Hypersomnia used by itself or in combination with other medicines.

Antihistamines will diminish the effects of pitolisant. Alternative treatments for the nasal congestion should be initiated, such as using a neti pot, Vicks VapoRub, menthol cough drops, over-the-counter nasal breathing strips, a humidifier, peppermint, nasal sprays, decongestants, or Singular (montelukast). If chronic allergies are a significant issue for the patient, and the above options are unsuccessful, an alternative medication or an ENT evaluation may need to be considered. Usually, this medicine can be tolerated unless their allergies are severe. Pitolisant, like others, can interfere with the effectiveness of hormonal birth control and will be discussed below. It can be used with alternative birth control methods, which must be continued for twenty-one days after discontinuing the medication.

Sunosi (solriamfetol): This medication is an FDA-approved treatment for Narcolepsy and the residual sleepiness of OSA. It is a dopamine and norepinephrine reuptake inhibitor. It has a dose-dependent effect, with higher doses leading to increased efficacy for EDS. It also has demonstrated early symptom improvement (Thorpy et al., 2019). Sunosi has none of the issues when taken with birth control pills that may be found with Nuvigil, Provigil, and Wakix. It can be associated with hypertension, and blood pressure should be monitored. Weaver and associates reported long-term improvement in quality of life and work productivity with EDS in OSA and Narcolepsy patients for up to fifty-two weeks (Weaver et al., 2021). Most recently, Van Dongen and associates reported that solriamfetol demonstrated improved cognitive performance in OSA patients (Van Dongen et al., 2023), which hopefully will be shown in Narcolepsy in future studies.

Antidepressants: Antidepressants, such as the Tricyclics and SSRI antidepressants, are REM suppressants and may help treat cataplexy, hypnogogic hallucination, sleep paralysis, insomnia, depression, and anxiety associated with Narcolepsy. Dr. Scammell's review reports the most robust clinical experience supports the efficacy of venlafaxine, but alternatives such as fluoxetine, duloxetine, protriptyline, and clomipramine have been used. Various other antidepressants have also been used over the years, especially where clinicians may be paying attention to any other co-existing disorders that may be present in addition to Narcolepsy and feel a specific antidepressant may be indicated. Side effects (such as sexual dysfunction), compliance issues, cost, drug interactions, and the prescribed medication time may also play in the decision. Reboxetine (an antidepressant used outside of the USA marketed as Edronax) has also been shown to help with cataplexy and excessive daytime sleepiness in Narcolepsy (Thorpy, 2020).

Miscellaneous Medications That Have Been Used for Narcolepsy

Strattera (atomoxetine) is a non-stimulant norepinephrine inhibitor used for ADHD. It was reported by Zhang and associates to improve excessive daytime sleepiness and cataplexy but had little effect on sleep paralysis or hypnogogic hallucinations (2015).

Early studies suggested Tegretol (carbamazepine) as a treatment for cataplexy (Vaughn & D'Cruz, 1996).

Selegiline (Eldepryl, Zelapa) has been used for cataplexy and EDS (Hublin et al., 1994). Still, it is not usually prescribed due to the high dosages required and the risk of dietary and medication interactions due to its chemical makeup as an MAO inhibitor (Abad & Guilleminault, 2017).

Baclofen has been reported to improve sleep quality in Narcolepsy by acting on what is known as GABA-B receptors. It has been shown to increase total sleep time and decrease wakefulness after sleep onset; others have reported it to help with excessive daytime sleepiness (Morse, Kelly-Pieper, & Kothare, 2019).

Future Treatment Options

In the "A narcotic-narcoleptic link" report (Bray, 2018), the author stated, "Hypothalamic neurons that produce hypocretin neuropeptides (also known as orexins) are involved in pleasure-associated arousal and have thus been hypothesized to have a role in opioid addiction." In Narcolepsy, about 90% of hypocretin cells are lost. A study by Thannickal and associates found human heroin addicts had 54% more hypocretin-producing neurons than neurologically normal individuals. They then explored the relationship between Narcolepsy, opioid addiction, and hypocretin cells and suggested that long-term opiate use might increase the number of hypothalamic hypocretin cells, decreasing symptoms of Narcolepsy such as cataplexy. They proposed this might "also explain previous reports that people with narcolepsy are resistant to drug addiction" (Thannickal et al., 2018).

A case report by Omari and Kinyungu (2022) revealed a 39-year-old female with Narcolepsy with cataplexy had decreased cataplexy after treatment with suboxone. These findings could be interesting for future therapies.

Mazindol is a partial orexin receptor agonist and triple monoamine reuptake inhibitor. It has been used for both excessive daytime sleepiness and cataplexy. It is a central nervous stimulant that increases alertness but has minimal effect on the cardiovascular system or mood. It is currently in Phase 2 studies in an extended-release form and was recently reported to decrease the number of weekly cataplexy episodes and improve daytime sleepiness (Bogan et al., 2023).

T-cell modifying medications are a newer class of drugs being considered, which includes natalizumab (Tysabri) (Scammell et al., 2020). This medicine was used based on the theory that Narcolepsy is due to autoimmune issues, and this medication inhibits T cells and other leukocytes from crossing the blood-brain barrier. This actual case study did not improve symptoms. Still, it was suggested that more extensive studies of T-cell modifying medications might be beneficial if started soon after the first symptoms of Narcolepsy.

General Medication Treatment Considerations

Next, I would like to discuss some general things we, as providers, consider when looking at treatment options for each Narcolepsy patient. If there is a way that we can treat two distinct symptoms/ disorders with one particular medication, simplification of the number of drugs prescribed is often the best option. For example, sodium oxybate and pitolisant are approved to treat both excessive daytime sleepiness and cataplexy in Narcolepsy and may be used as a single agent to treat Narcolepsy. As I said, I use them all, and combinations of meds or layering of medications are used most often. Usually, I give patients PRN meds they can use as required, as medication needs vary based on their daily tasks, sleep the night before, the weather, and other health issues.

The following are some very general guidelines when considering medications:

Are they already on antidepressants? These meds can be partially or fully treating cataplexy. This needs to be considered while establishing the diagnosis. A patient who may have been on antidepressants for several years may not have current symptoms of cataplexy as the antidepressants would have suppressed the cataplexy. This may prevent the diagnosis of type 1 Narcolepsy with cataplexy. Looking back to their history before starting antidepressants or when antidepressants may have been forgotten can help distinguish these symptoms. Alternatively, when considering treatment if the patient is suffering from depression and or anxiety in addition to their symptoms of Narcolepsy with cataplexy, switching to antidepressants may help "kill two birds with one stone." Or, if possible, they may need a higher dose of the antidepressant to treat both symptoms.

Co-occurring Obstructive Sleep Apnea and Narcolepsy in patients. If patients have both Obstructive Sleep Apnea and Narcolepsy, in addition to using the CPAP, Sunosi (solriameftol), Provigil (modafinil), and Nuvigil (armodafinil) have all been FDA-approved to treat EDS in both disorders. The patient **must** be using CPAP if on the oxybates.

Evaluation of the patient's other medications. Are they on sedating meds? What time of the day are they taking their medications? We may need to adjust the timing of multiple meds or consider switching medication in patients taking sedating meds that could cause EDS, like blood pressure meds, sedating antidepressants, and allergy meds.

In patients with co-existing ADHD, stimulants may be able to treat both disorders. Usually, a combination of both a long-acting stimulant and a PRN of a short-acting stimulant is required. The long-acting medication Journay PM may be helpful for those Narcolepsy patients having both conditions and significant sleep inertia.

In patients with hypertension or other cardiac issues, we consider the side effects of sodium oxybate, solriameftol, and stimulants. Pitolisant doses should be decreased with other medications that cause **cardiac conduction delays** and avoided in those with a history of cardiac arrhythmias. It is suggested that the oxybate dose be decreased by half in those with hepatic impairment.

With hepatic or renal failure, several medications may cause issues. Wakix (pitolisant) is contraindicated in patients with severe hepatic impairment and not recommended in patients with end-stage renal disease. It requires adjustment in dosing in those with moderate hepatic or renal impairment. Sunosi (solriameftol) is not recommended in patients with end-stage renal disease. The oxybates have a high salt intake, which should be considered with renal impairment. The lower sodium Xywav may be a consideration. Nuvigil (armodafinil) and Provigil (modafinil) should be used cautiously in severe renal impairment, and their dose should be decreased by half with hepatic impairment.

Do they drink alcohol? We avoid oxybates in patients if they use alcohol more than on very rare occasions (birthdays or holidays). If they consume alcohol only on special events, patients can use the alcohol but can NOT take the Xyrem/Xywav/Lumryz on the nights they use any alcohol—at all! If they use alcohol more regularly, Xyrem, Xywav, or Lumryz would not be an appropriate medication.

Does the patient have a lot of disrupted nocturnal sleep? If so, Xyrem, Xywav, or Lumryz could be an effective treatment option for excessive daytime sleepiness, cataplexy, and disrupted nocturnal sleep. If insomnia and disrupted nocturnal sleep are significant issues, we avoid late-day stimulants, longer-acting stimulants, or activating antidepressants. Patients should also ensure they take their Provigil (modafinil), Nuvigil (armodafinil), Wakix (pitolisant), or Sunosi (solriamfetol) early enough in the day to prevent insomnia. Some more sedating antidepressants and other sleeping medications can be helpful, but not in combination with oxybates (see Chapter 3). One significant insomnia-related issue is that patients with Narcolepsy cannot take Quvivq (daridorexant), as it can worsen the symptoms of Narcolepsy!

Patients with co-existing anxiety. In this case, we avoid stimulants, use lower doses or less activating stimulants, or prescribe something like Wakix (pitolisant), Provigil (modafinil), or Nuvigil (armodafinil). If the anxiety is a significant source of stress and possibly contributes to cataplexy, an antidepressant, less sedating anxiety medication, pitolisant, or Xyrem/Xywav/Lumryz may be necessary (although there is a risk of anxiety as a side effect of Xyrem/Xywav/Lumryz).

What if the patient lives in a college dorm/apartment? In situations where there are many people in and out of the rooms, or the patient is living in a house with a known substance abuser or individuals struggling with substance use, we must consider the risks of having Xyrem, Xywav, or Lumryz, and stimulants in the home. At the very least, these medications should be locked in a safe and sometimes must be avoided altogether.

What if the patient has a history of substance abuse issues in the past? Some treatment choices may be limited for those with a history of substance abuse. Wakix is a non-controlled option. But there are still many options, such as antidepressants. The prior substance abuse may have also been to self-medicate undiagnosed Narcolepsy signs and symptoms, which must also be considered.

Narcolepsy Treatment and Birth Control

Modafinil, armodafinil, and pitolisant are all medications that could interfere with the effectiveness of birth control pills. With the risk of sexually transmitted diseases, some patients already use other birth control options to decrease their exposure to STD risk. Regardless, alternatives should be considered, such as Sunosi or other medications without effects on birth control, using an IUD, condoms, a birth control pill with higher levels of hormones, or a combination thereof. I have found that many people do not shy away from modafinil, armodafinil, and pitolisant and use additional levels of protection. Additionally, you must remember to use alternative forms of birth control for at least twenty-one days after stopping pitolisant.

Family and Peer Support

Be open and willing to accept social support. Let others support you and teach them how to do it well by giving specific recommendations. Educate your family, friends, school, work, and community on the specifics of Narcolepsy. Share this book and Julie Flygare's book. Please direct them to Project Sleep, Wake Up Narcolepsy, the Narcolepsy Network, and their support groups. Do individual therapy to discuss your issues and define your needs and consider family therapy to discuss the consequences of this illness on you and your family. It does change things. Attend support groups online or in person. Peer support is an amazing resource! Multiple support groups online are available at the websites mentioned above.

"I cannot stress enough how important it is to find a like-minded tribe who believes in you so ferociously that on the days you feel like you can't, they remind you that YOU CAN."
@ninaslostandfound I MW Facets

From: "Knock Out Depression" Facebook page

I saw this on Pinterest (and on *The Mighty*) and feel it is very appropriate here:

"I am constantly torn between: I can't let this illness ruin my life, and I have to listen to my body and rest."

There is no easy answer to that question. And it will vary from time to time. Be willing to set limits, but don't exclude yourself from activities or family memories. Give your loved one's grace—this journey probably took you a long time to discover. Your family and friends may want to help but often try to fix it with "just do this . . ." Explore options together. Let them help with the problem-solving as necessary. When something is significant to them, you may need to work to find a way around your sleepiness or other symptoms to be a part of that activity or function. The journey and discovering your path can help build the relationship. Communication is vital, and isolation is not necessary or beneficial.

Sleep Hygiene and Behavioral Treatments for Insomnia

We all hear about sleep hygiene and recommend it for various disorders associated with insomnia. Let me give you some of the more specific recommendations we use for sleep hygiene:

- Three to four hours before bedtime, reduce fluids to prevent waking to go to the bathroom during sleep if that is an issue.
- Avoid alcohol at least three to four hours or more before bedtime. Alcohol really can be disruptive to sleep and increase sleep apnea if present. While it may initially help some people get to sleep, it disrupts sleep quality, and tolerance can build, requiring higher amounts of alcohol to even help with sleep promotion. It can also increase bathroom trips.
- Stop caffeine after 3:00 p.m.
- Avoid nicotine before bedtime, and do not smoke if you wake up in the middle of the night. Nicotine is a stimulant and can delay sleep onset and cause disruptions during sleep. Smoking can decrease the quality of sleep as well as the quantity of sleep.
- Avoid evening naps. A short catnap immediately after school or work may be okay. Do not take long naps (one to two hours) in the evenings.
- If taking stimulants, avoid after 4:00 p.m. and use only short-acting stimulants in the afternoon or evening.

- Exercise during the day is helpful, but not within three to four hours of sleep.
- Do not eat heavy meals before bedtime. Eat dinner earlier and have a light snack before bedtime if needed.
- Treat gastroesophageal reflux disease symptoms if present and use positional therapy to decrease the severity.
- Start to dim the lights and lower the volume of TV shows or music one to two hours before sleep. Avoid bright lights in the evening and overstimulation.
- Epsom salt soaks may be helpful to ease chronic pain, reduce stress, release muscle tension, and decrease restless legs symptoms. It should be avoided if pregnant, in those with significantly dry skin, and possibly with diabetes.
- Schedule a sleep time that allows you to get seven to eight hours of sleep and start to prepare for bed at least an hour before your desired bedtime. This can be accomplished by taking a hot shower or bath, avoiding the news or action shows on the television, turning off electronics, listening to relaxing music, making a bedtime music playlist, doing some light stretching, not having emotionally stimulating conversations or paying bills late at night, considering using lavender or other essential oil, meditating, have sex or cuddle time with your partner, praying, exhaling, and practicing progressive relaxation or imagery visualization.
- Progressive muscle relaxation involves slowing down your breathing, giving yourself permission to relax, then slowly tensing for 10–15 seconds, then relaxing for about thirty seconds, all of your muscle groups starting with your toes and working your way up to your head. Then, imagine releasing all the worries, thoughts, and concerns trapped in your brain.
- Guided imagery or imagery visualization involves using your mind and imagination to envision yourself more relaxed in an imagined scene or situation. While imagining this

scene or situation, you allow your memory to visualize as many of the details of the location as you can, imagine the smells and sounds from the scene, any sense of touch you might feel in that situation, and even taste, if it is part of your visualization. There are websites and audio files with verbal directions you may listen to lead you through progressive muscle relaxation and guided imagery if you desire a more formalized approach.

- Make sure your bedroom and your bed are comforting, relaxing, and free of chaos. Do not work in bed. Use a noise machine if there is environmental noise that would disrupt your sleep. Make sure the temperature is cool and not too hot or cold. Make sure your mattress and pillow are both comfortable and supportive. Ensure there is not too much outside light that would prevent sleep. Room darkening curtains, using cut-out cardboard or even aluminum foil applied to the inside of the window to block outside light may help to avoid disruption. Remove clutter from the bed. Do not sleep with your pets or kids, if possible; they are often a significant source of sleep disruption. If your bed partner snores, ask them to be evaluated. Alternatively, you may need to sleep in another room if their snoring is significant.
- Keep your schedule consistent. Go to bed and get up at about the same time every day.
- Go to bed only when sleepy and get back up if you are not asleep in twenty minutes. Do some non-stimulating activity (examples include looking at a magazine, folding laundry, watching a comedy or light-hearted show, listening to music, but do NOT get on electronics, watch the news, start a movie, or watch an action-packed show, drama, or cop show). Return to bed when you are relaxed and sleepy.
- Use your bed for sleep, naps, and sex only. Do not hang out in bed during the day or several hours before your

desired sleep time. Your body and mind will not associate your bed with sleep.

- My friend, distinguished colleague, and sleep doctor to many professional sporting teams, W. Chris Winter MD, has written a very readable, user-friendly book for insomnia, including a section on Narcolepsy and insomnia called *The Sleep Solution*. I suggest you consider reading this too! I often recommend his book to my patients.

Other Behavioral Treatments of Narcolepsy

(Marín Agudelo et al., 2014) (A. M. Morse, 2019)

- Light therapy and sunlight can help. Get outside, get fresh air, get sunshine, and get moving!
- Aromatherapy. Use rosemary to alert, as well as lemon, orange, grapefruit, clove, basil, cinnamon, and peppermint. Lavender is best to relax and aid with sleep.
- Plan appointments and car trips based on your daily sleepiness symptoms.
- Yoga can improve sleep by focusing breathing and attention on physical movements. Combining mindfulness, breathing regulation, stretching, and physical activity can lead to physical and mental relaxation and overall wellness.
- Keep a regular sleep schedule. Avoid long sleep-ins, get up, get dressed, and make the bed.
- Alarm clocks. Vibrating alarm clocks with gradual light therapy, two or three alarm clocks across the room, and a "sonic boom" alarm clock may be necessary. There is a wide variety of these available to purchase online.

Sometimes, for patients having great trouble waking up in the morning, we advise them to set one alarm to wake about one hour before their required time to get up and take a short-acting stimulant. They can keep this medication beside their bed and only need to rise briefly to swallow it. The short-acting stimulant will then have time to get into the system, allowing patients to be more alert and have an easier time getting up, when necessary, when their second alarm goes off. Alternatively, a stimulant like Journay PM (methylphenidate HCL extended release) can be taken at night and may be helpful for sleepiness in the morning in those having ADHD and co-existing Narcolepsy.

Therapy/Counseling

- Individual/family therapy, group therapy for Narcolepsy, and groups on the Internet are priceless. I cannot emphasize enough the power of supportive peer groups in treating Narcolepsy!
- Cognitive behavioral therapy for insomnia, hypersomnia, cataplexy, depression, and anxiety are helpful interventions for Narcolepsy. Other options for insomnia include smartphone apps such as the "CBT-I Coach," a forehead temperature cooling device, and mindfulness training with CBT-I (Rosenberg et al., 2021).
- Imagery rehearsal therapy for nightmares can be beneficial, and this will be discussed in more detail later in this chapter.
- Hypnosis has been reported to help with sleep paralysis and sleepiness.

Dietary Accommodations

- Various dietary changes have been recommended to assist. Look for what influences or helps you the most.
- Small, frequent meals with healthy snacks instead of large meals may be of benefit.

- A ketogenic diet, restricting carbohydrates to 10–15 mg, a 1-gram protein diet, and the Atkins Diet have all been reported by some patients to be of benefit. Others have also suggested gluten-free diets as being helpful. High carbohydrate diets often make even people without Narcolepsy sleepy.
- Look for food intolerances, including chocolate, alcohol, and turkey, as causes of increased sedation or other symptoms. Look for things that worsen your sleepiness, such as heavy meals, late meals, or sweets.
- Look for something that worsens your anxiety, such as excessive caffeine or decongestants, and avoid those.
- Caffeine and alcohol may also contribute to insomnia, contributing to the cycle of hypersomnia and insomnia seen with Narcolepsy.

Nutritional Supplements

- Magnesium has been used for insomnia, nocturnal leg cramps, pain/stiffness, and restless legs and is reported to improve sleep quality and duration. It should be avoided during pregnancy until discussed with the OB/GYN.
- Melatonin has been used as a supplement for insomnia but can lead to vivid dreams. It has been suggested that melatonin can improve insomnia and hypersomnolence by altering sleep architecture and improving REM sleep abnormalities (Xie et al., 2017).

Lifestyle Changes

- Try relaxation techniques. A grounding technique used for anxiety involves the "5, 4, 3, 2, 1" approach in which you take a few moments to search for five things you can see, four things you can touch, three things you can hear, two things you can smell, and one thing you can taste. (Keep gum, mints, or licorice with you.)

- Breathing techniques that can help include putting a hand on your chest and one on your abdomen and noticing that you are breathing and moving your stomach more than your chest as you slow your breathing down. Then, try breathing in through your nose and out through your mouth. Practice inhaling for a count of five, holding your breath for a count of five, and then exhaling to a count of five. People use different numbers for this exercise, often with a longer exhale time. The point is to notice your breathing, breathe more from your abdomen, slow your breathing down, and exhale to relax.

- Manage safety concerns. Avoid driving, climbing, swimming, cooking, or other dangerous activities when sleepy or having cataplexy.

- Avoid hot environments that might make you sleepy. The cooler, the better.

- Say no and don't feel guilty. Those who love you will understand when you can't go out. Know your limits. But remember, they have feelings, too, and you must recognize and validate their feelings as well! Sometimes, you may have to go sleepy or grab a 15-minute strategic nap before going.

- Get "Rest **and** Relaxation," not just sleep. Work on self-care. Schedule downtime and time just hanging out with your family and friends. It cannot all be about your Narcolepsy, naps, and sleep. Life is short. Enjoy! Have fun! Start a hobby, craft, write, take pictures, play music, take walks, go hiking, enjoy nature, celebrate the sun, marvel at the moon and the stars, call an old friend, daydream, plan a date with your partner, and celebrate life! You are not your Narcolepsy! You are a person with Narcolepsy and deserve fun and to live life to the fullest!

- Avoid triggers at specific times but don't try to avoid all emotions all the time! For example, if laughter is one of the precipitants of cataplexy, advise your friends and family members not to tell jokes while you are walking down the stairs, driving, or during other activities that may be dangerous for you. But don't stop laughing and having fun when sitting or in a safe environment.
- Alert others. I suggest patients wear an identification badge or bracelet that can be worn to alert others if you have an episode of cataplexy or are found asleep. Have a way to warn others of what is happening and what they should or should not do. Bracelets can be ordered online, or we have created a medical badge you can order at the back of the book. Patients with Narcolepsy who drive also need signs to put in their car windows if they have a habit of napping in the car at lunchtime, before going home from work, or if they have to pull over on a driving trip. Nowadays, anyone seen sleeping in their vehicle is assumed to be a drug-related incident or overdose, and much excitement may be initiated to alert someone of this possibility and bring on the Narcan! We also have an offer for one of these windshield/school/workplace cards in the back of the book and will discuss this more below under driving with Narcolepsy.
- School and work modifications are discussed more in Chapter 11.

Other Options

- Meditation. There are many options for practicing meditation these days. YouTube videos, DVDs, audio recordings, apps, yoga classes, and therapy sessions are just a few options. I recently recorded an audio topic on Obstructive Sleep Apnea for the *5 Minutes For Me* app, with hopes to do a brief one on Narcolepsy in the future. The *5 Minutes For Me* app has meditations of five, ten, and twenty minutes, along with audio recordings on various topics such as wellness, mindset, resilience, self-help, and productivity. There are multiple resources for meditation on the Internet.

- Practice gratitude and mindfulness. Be grateful for the things you can do. Keep a gratitude journal. Focus on your abilities, not your disabilities, with Narcolepsy.
- Create a playlist, one to get you moving when sleepy and one to help you wind down and relax during the evening. You may also want to create one for when you feel discouraged, which may be more motivating and uplifting. Also consider one for when you are driving, which would be energizing and alerting.

For Brain Fog/Concentration Issues

We want patients to feel awake, alert, aware, concentrating well, and cognitively clear! The "brain fog" is an important but often overlooked symptom of Narcolepsy. If this symptom is present, this may be a place where a stimulant could help with both EDS and concentration.

Other options include:

- Writing things down.
- Using a recorder or Dictaphone.
- Dictating things into the Microsoft Word processing program.
- Use the Microsoft Word Read Aloud program or have something read to you with other reading apps if you struggle with concentration.

- Choose your most alert times to work on tasks requiring significant concentration. Try to be in an area free of distractions and sit up.
- Over the years, aromatherapy has also been suggested to improve concentration, using oils such as rosemary, cinnamon, sage, and peppermint.

Napping is Necessary!

"Naps! Naps! Naps! There is a nap for that!" As Dr. Richard Bogan said in a lecture he gave, "You must plan for that." In various parts of the world, such as Spain and Japan, napping at lunch is normal, protected, and increases productivity. We should consider this more seriously.

- Napping is not a luxury when you have Narcolepsy; it is a necessity!
- Naps should usually be 10–30 minutes long (at most) and scheduled to precede times when the patient has the most difficulty staying awake.
- A single long nap of about 120 minutes has been reported to be helpful in some instead of several short naps, but the effect may wear off in about three hours.
- Keep to a regular bedtime and good sleep hygiene. Avoid sleep deprivation.

Time your naps during the time of day for when you are the sleepiest. One of the benefits of the NAPS screener we created was to ask patients specifically about their degree of sleepiness in the morning (8:00 a.m. to noon), afternoon (noon to 6:00 p.m.), and evening (6:00 p.m. to 10:00 p.m.). We have found this helps us tailor meds to the various times of the day and naps to the times most needed. Even a brief nap after work or school may make the evenings much more tolerable for the patient, their family, evening social activities, and household chores. But I also must caution you not to allow naps to rule you. Regularly scheduled routine naps are helpful; being rigid about your naps can limit you. And napping too long in the evening can be disruptive to nighttime sleep.

Treatment of Nightmares and Vivid Dreams

Vivid dreams and nightmares are usually part of the REM-related symptoms found with Narcolepsy. They can be so disruptive that people are afraid to sleep at night and afraid to schedule and take restorative daytime naps. The nightmares can be treated in a variety of ways. Medications and cognitive-based therapies are used, such as imagery rehearsal therapy (IRT) and exposure, relaxation, and rescripting therapy (ERRT). Imagery rehearsal therapy (Krakow et al., 1995) has the patient create alternate endings to their reoccurring nightmares that are nonfrightening and rehearse the dreams with a new ending. Exposure, relaxation, and rescription therapy (Davis & Wright, 2006) uses psychoeducation about nightmares, sleep hygiene, relaxation training, and nightmare exposure and rescripting. Medications that have been used to treat nightmares are prazosin, triazolam, olanzapine, risperidone, aripiprazole, clonidine, cyproheptadine, gabapentin, fluvoxamine, nabilone, topiramate, trazodone, and tricyclic antidepressants (Morgenthaler et al., 2018). Although prazosin is frequently used for nightmares, there have been occasional reports that it may increase cataplexy.

I listened to an interview with Barry Krakow, MD, on *The Carlat Psychiatry Podcast* on "Why Nightmares Matter" (8/22/2021), where he suggested asking patients if they thought about their nightmare content during the day. He also advised looking to evaluate for sleep apnea as nightmares are a sign of sleep apnea. He helped to develop the behavioral therapy for nightmares called imagery rehearsal therapy. You can find out more information on his website, barrykrakowmd.com.

Some experts report sleeping in a room that is too hot can lead to nightmares and night terrors, and sleeping in cooler temperatures may be helpful. Sleep deprivation is another reason for nightmares, as you have REM rebound sleep, leading to increased dreaming and possibly nightmares. So, once again, keep your sleep schedule regular!

REM Sleep Behavior Disorder

Another REM-related sleep issue associated with Narcolepsy is REM Sleep Behavior Disorder. This finding is sometimes seen in the pediatric and adult populations with Narcolepsy. As you may recall, REM Sleep Behavior Disorder is acting out of dreams while asleep with kicking, punching, yelling, etc. Clonazepam is probably the most frequently used treatment for this disorder. Other medications that have been used include melatonin, pramipexole, temazepam, donepezil, lorazepam, zolpidem, zopiclone, ramelteon, agomelatine, cannabinoids, and sodium oxybate, as well as a bed alarm system (Jung & St. Louis, 2016). Behavioral treatments are also essential to prevent injury if this disorder is more severe, such as moving furniture around in the bedroom or even out of the room to avoid injury, removing dangerous objects out of close reach in the bedroom (guns, knives, baseball bats), applying padding to furniture, protecting the windows with shatterproof glass or padding, and if necessary, have the bed partner sleep in another room.

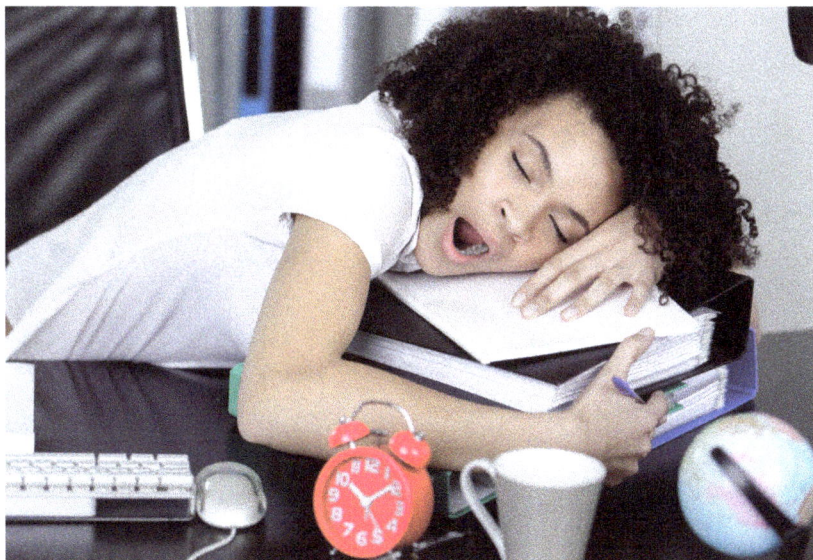

Get More Knowledge!

Here are some further resources where you can learn more:

Ted Talks:

- TED Talk by Angie Collins, "Purpose(fully) Living With Narcolepsy," May 29, 2015, with her brain "channel surfing" on its own
- TED Talk by Julie Flyger, "What Can You Learn From A Professional Dreamer?" July 13, 2022
- TED Talk by Maeve Sheehy, "The Power of a Disability," Feb 27, 2017
- TED Talk by Lum-Awah Atang Arrey, "Lessons From Narcolepsy: How to Snooze and Not Lose," Dec 20, 2022.

YouTube Videos:

- "Living with Narcolepsy" from Harvard Medical School, Feb 21, 2014
- "Everyone with Narcolepsy Has a Different Story to Tell" Feb 28, 2020
- "Diagnosing Narcolepsy" with Dr. Kiran Maski from Harvard Medical School, Feb 21, 2014
- "Behind the Mystery: Narcolepsy" The Balancing Act, Oct 30, 2018
- "What Is Narcolepsy and What to Do About It" Dr. Tracey Marks, Jan 24, 2018
- "Behavioral Treatments for Narcolepsy" by Dr. Ariel Neikrug, Jan 31, 2022;
- "Cognitive Behavioral Therapy In Insomnia" Karl Doghramji, MD, Aug 22, 2019

Sleepiness, Safety, and Driving with Narcolepsy

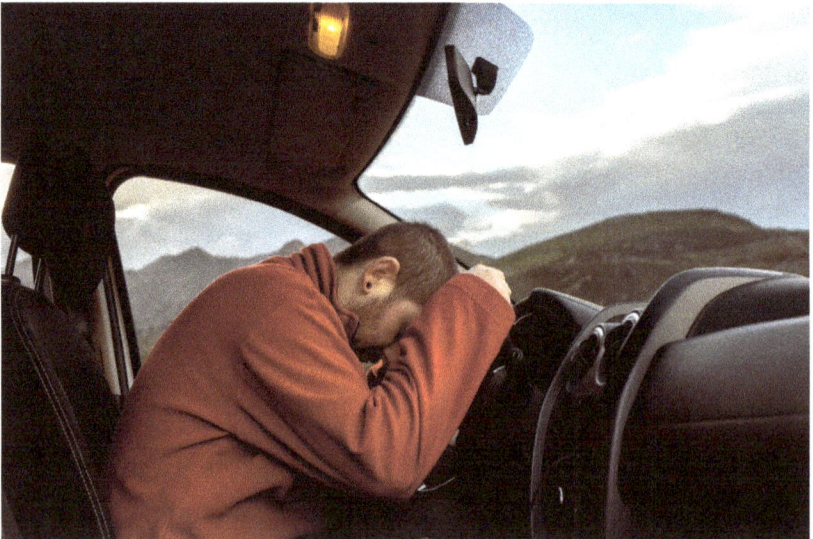

Unless you are treated for your Narcolepsy, don't drive. It would be too dangerous. With the appropriate treatment and stabilization of symptoms, some people with Narcolepsy can drive. Ensure your excessive daytime sleepiness and cataplexy symptoms are well controlled. Don't drive when sleepy, or immediately pull over if you get tired while driving! If you have severe Narcolepsy, the best option is not to drive. You should plan to drive around times when you are usually most alert. It may be that the timing of your medications needs to be about one hour before your driving time or that you have a PRN of a stimulant to use at least one hour before driving if suffering from significant hypersomnia. You may need to find a quiet area to nap before you drive home from work or school. Other options include taking an Uber/taxi, ride share, the shuttle, the bus, living near campus/work, and walking. For those driving, I suggest you have a "Therapeutic Nap In Progress" plaque you put in the window while napping (I have an offer for one of these car cards in the back of the book). Nowadays, anyone seen sleeping in their vehicle is assumed to be a drug-related incident or overdose, and much excitement may be initiated to alert someone.

Drive during the day when you can. Use sunglasses and your visor to avoid the bright sunlight shining in your eyes while driving. Use wetting eye drops if dry eyes contribute at all to your feelings of sleepiness. Keep upbeat music playing. Make a driving playlist to energize you and help you stay awake. Talk with someone you know while you are driving to keep alert. Never drink and drive! Avoid heavy meals or sweets before going. Use caffeine if it is early enough in the day. Keep trips as short as possible and take a break at least every one to two hours if driving long distances. If possible, don't drive alone. Keep your sleep schedule regular and avoid driving if sleep deprived. Take a power nap before you go. Do not take allergy medications or new over-the-counter medicines before you drive. You may not realize they could contribute to sleepy driving.

States have various reporting standards regarding driving with Narcolepsy. The National Highway Traffic Safety Administration allows people with Narcolepsy to drive if they receive treatment. Still, some states like Pennsylvania and California require you to report conditions like Narcolepsy. Be sure to check with your specific state before driving. Regardless of the requirements, we sometimes must report to the authorities patients known to be non-compliant. I once had to report a patient with Obstructive Sleep Apnea and Narcolepsy who was non-compliant with his CPAP and medications for both of these disorders and got a job as a school bus driver!

The danger of this was highlighted for me when one of my patients being treated for significant Narcolepsy told me he felt his Father may have had undiagnosed Narcolepsy as he had five severe car wrecks—one that ultimately killed him. When in doubt, the answer is always don't drive!

I do not automatically take the license of someone diagnosed with Narcolepsy. A lot of variables play into that decision. If compliant with treatment and symptoms are controlled, I will use PRN stimulants if the patient is having a significantly sleepy day. If the patient is non-compliant and we have not adequately controlled the symptoms, I do not allow patients to drive until stabilized. If pushed, I will report them if I feel there is a danger to the patient or others. I recommend patients pull over and nap, use a PRN stimulant, and call someone to get them if sleepiness becomes even moderately significant. I advise them to be aware of their signs of increased sleepiness, such as increased yawning, head bobbing, when their eyes feel very heavy, difficulty concentrating on the road, and if they find themselves swerving, crossing midline, or going off the side of the road. I instruct them to rate their sleepiness on a scale of one to ten before they start to drive, with ten being the sleepiest. If their value is five or over, they should probably not drive. If this value starts to increase while they are driving, they should immediately pull over.

The Hypersomnia Foundation website has good information about safely sleeping/napping in your car. I suggest you look at it.

Narcolepsy, Sleepiness, and Smoking

- Go outside to smoke. Don't risk falling asleep while smoking in your house.
- Stand up to smoke.
- Have someone with you when you smoke.
- Better yet, don't smoke! (Sorry, I couldn't avoid inserting my opinion here.)

Chapter 6

The Sleepy Child

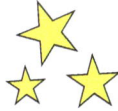

⭐⭐⭐

Pediatric and Adolescent Narcolepsy

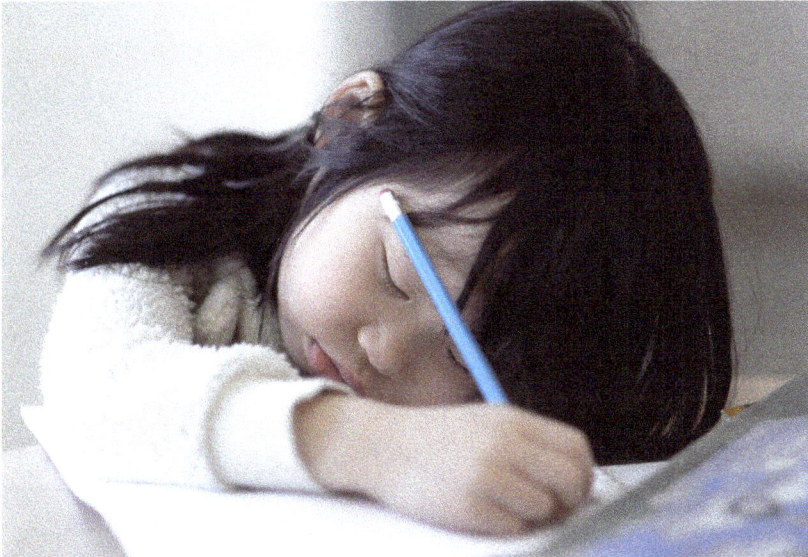

*"Without enough sleep, we all become tall
two-year-olds."*
JoJo Jensen

Let's return to discussing children who may present with increased irritability, frustration, confusion, bewilderment, school failure, and isolation. And they may feel "everybody is always mad at me." The excessive daytime sleepiness of Narcolepsy often presents in childhood and adolescence but is not recognized or diagnosed until much later. The Nexus Narcolepsy Registry (Ohayon et al., 2021) data indicate that Narcolepsy symptoms commonly manifest during childhood/adolescence, with a median onset of 16 years of age and a substantial average delay from symptom onset to Narcolepsy diagnosis of 11.8 years. Let's help decrease that delay!

Children and adolescents require much more sleep than they usually get. Children need at least nine to eleven hours of sleep, and adolescents need about eight to ten hours. Do you know any teenagers who actually get that much sleep each night? They may have extended naps after school, but their nighttime sleep is often disrupted. High school students are especially sleep-deprived with many after-school activities, delayed sleep schedules, late-night electronic use, homework demands, and early rise times. There are many movements to change school start times to help address this issue. Having a disorder of Narcolepsy in addition to these issues is especially significant. Sleepiness is assumed to be due to the abovementioned problems, and Narcolepsy may be overlooked.

Sometimes, teachers may be the first to realize the child/adolescent patient appears sleepy and is not getting enough sleep. Alternatively, their lack of attention, trouble with assignments, seeming to "daze off" with microsleeps, missing assignments, and falling asleep at school may be diagnosed as ADHD, laziness, poor motivation, substance abuse, depression, and irritability. Many children and adolescents with Narcolepsy are misdiagnosed with ADHD and prescribed stimulants, which actually may help them with their sleepiness and "brain fog." Also, ADHD and Narcolepsy can coexist

(A. Morse & Sanjeev, 2018). Additionally, Narcolepsy can also be labeled as depression.

> *"Let's start by taking a smallish nap . . . or two."*
>
> *Winnie the Pooh*

Naps in children usually stop around five to six years of age but can reemerge in Narcolepsy. Younger children may not have the words to describe Narcolepsy symptoms, and their parents may notice unusual behavior, facial grimacing, or behavioral complaints. This may hint that something is wrong, and vague symptoms may be reported to their pediatrician. We must alert others to Narcolepsy as a potential issue when these symptoms are present. I was doing a talk on Narcolepsy once, where a pediatric neurologist nearing the end of her career said she may have seen only one case of Narcolepsy throughout her many years of neurology. I realized she may not have been aware of the subtle ways Narcolepsy can present and may have sometimes missed this diagnosis. Our knowledge about Narcolepsy is advancing rapidly. We need to ensure pediatricians, family practitioners, psychiatrists, neurologists, physician assistants, nurse practitioners, therapists, drug reps, and the school system (teachers and school counselors) know how Narcolepsy may present in the pediatric and adolescent population.

Sleepiness in child and adolescent patients can be evaluated using the Epworth Sleepiness Scale for Children and Adolescents (ESS-CHAD)(Wang et al., 2017), a sleep diary, a cataplexy diary, the Pediatric Daytime Sleepiness Scale (Drake et al., 2003), the Pediatric Hypersomnolence Survey (Maski et al., 2022) and others (Benmedjahed et al., 2017). Of course, the PSG/MSLT is also necessary. At the back of this book, I have included our recently developed Pediatric Narcolepsy Assessment & Progress Screener (Stultz, Kass,

& Herpel, 2023). This screener includes questions about sleepiness and sleep schedules, screens for school difficulties, assesses for all the Narcolepsy symptoms, lists possible cataplexy presentations, and asks the parents to list treatment goals.

In the book *Narcolepsy*, Thorpy (2016a, p.47–49) described pediatric Narcolepsy in the following way:

"In children, the patient may have an increased amount of sleep in a 24-hour period, and the sleepiness may vary from day to day, but they are never free of it; they may have 'automatic behavior' where they can appear like they are awake with no recall for the activity; and cataplexy in children may be more likely to be precipitated by negative emotions, such as anger. It can be precipitated by stress, exhaustion, or feeling tired. Children are often described as having 'puppet-like movements,' which can progress into cataplexy. Hypnogogic hallucinations, vivid dreams, nightmares, lucid dreams, and sleep paralysis may occur. Delusional dreams in which the patient actually believes what they dreamed can be present. School-aged children may have 'nap attacks' with irresistible urges to sleep. Sleepiness in children may be associated with the re-emergence of napping, longer naps, and naps that might not be refreshing. Their tiredness may contribute to poor academic performance and cognitive dysfunction, and they may have more irritability and behavioral problems. Teachers can be beneficial at identifying sleepiness in school, but the child is often described as 'lazy' and 'not paying attention in school.' Some social consequences may be present with poor peer interactions."

There are many videos found online that I feel may be helpful for you to review when considering pediatric/adolescent Narcolepsy issues, such as:

- "A violent call to sleep" https://youtu.be/KinZiCVEISM
- "Diagnosing Narcolepsy" Harvard Medical School: https://youtu.be/ZiPPqNh1jzg
- "Narcolepsy simply explained for Kids": https://youtu.be/H2cUg6H2h7Q

Cataplexy in Children and Adolescents

There are many different descriptions of cataplexy in children, and the pediatric presentation of cataplexy may appear much different from that of the adult population. The cataplexy may evolve over time and become more like the adult presentation as children age. Children may have an atypical presentation without an emotional trigger and with "cataplectic facies" (Anic-Labat et al., 1999b). Anic-Labat and associates reported the face or neck muscles were more involved than the limbs, and cataplexy was best differentiated from other muscle weaknesses when triggered by hearing and telling a joke, while laughing, and when angry. According to Serra and associates (Serra et al., 2008a), children can have muscle atonia without an emotional trigger, which may present with tongue thrusting and jaw weakness. Their article has a good picture of "cataplectic facies" in a child watching a cartoon. Cataplexy may be more severe and prolonged in the prepubertal child and might be associated with decreased muscle tone, prominent facial or jaw weakness, eyelid weakness, spontaneous tongue protrusion, neck extension, slurred speech, grimacing, self-scratching, and touching (Plazzi et al., 2018).

In another study, Pillen and associates described a complex movement disorder around the onset in kids, with repetitive tongue movements or thrusting, raising eyebrows, grimacing, lip chewing, loss of muscle tone in the face, and head bobbing due to neck weakness (Pillen et al., 2017). The head drop, facial hypotonia, drooping eyelids, and almost Down's-like tongue protrusion are often called "negative" motor features, with the lip chewing, tongue thrusting, mouth repeatedly opening with chewing-like activity, and raising eyebrows being called "active" movements.

Some online videos of cataplexy in the pediatric/adolescent population are as follows:

- "This is Cataplexy," Lanna Barrison, Jan 22, 2018: https://youtu.be/OaB9Ss3AZew
- "I like to make Dylan laugh, but It makes him fall," Sylvia Barrison-Scott: www.wakeupDylan.com
- "Cataplexy is so stupid, and it's not faired!" by Dylan Barrison: www.wakeupDylan.com
- "Narcolepsy in Very Young Children: A Parents' Perspective" by Lanna Barrison, 2019, Pediatric Sleep Conference: https://youtu.be/nfsLUlp3sxl
- "Cataplexy Attack," SierraJade220: https://youtu.be/VA6FeiGgLF0
- "Teen Suffering From Narcolepsy Sleep Up to 10 Times A Day": https://youtu.be/rQWG9d7ReYs
- "Narcolepsy simply explained for Kids" by Lanna Barrison: https://youtu.be/H2cUg6H2h7Q.
- "Faces of Narcolepsy": https://youtu.be/KinZiCVEISM
- "Diagnosing Narcolepsy," Harvard Medical School: https://youtu.be/ZiPPqNh1jzg

Lanna Barrison, in her slides from her YouTube presentation "Narcolepsy in Very Young Children," reported, "Fun=Cataplexy." This statement brings up a key point about cataplexy. Patients often learn at an incredibly early age that laughter or other strong emotions are associated with cataplexy, and they may seek to avoid this symptom and strong feelings to prevent cataplexy and avoid embarrassment. Due to this, they may avoid parties, sporting activities, sleepovers,

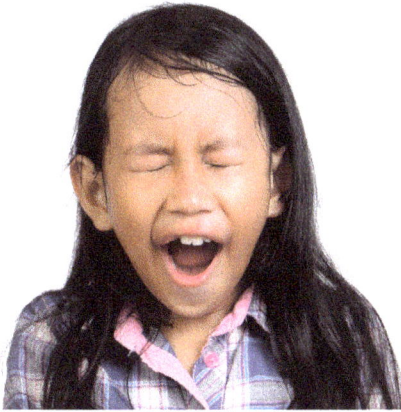

and other appropriate age-related activities, leading to social isolation, depression, and delayed social and sexual development. This finding should not be overlooked in the adult population with cataplexy as well.

In the Harvard Medical School YouTube video "Diagnosing Narcolepsy," Dr. Kiran Maski is working with an adolescent patient whose Mother described her daughter as "really upbeat, high energy, and her symptoms of sleepiness are out of character with her personality and her level of outgoingness." This presentation is an excellent example of how a patient may be misdiagnosed as having depression, laziness, or even hormonal issues because they appear so different after the onset of Narcolepsy symptoms.

Kids with Narcolepsy may be unfairly labeled "bad kids" by educators. Teixeira and associates (2004) interviewed forty-five adult patients with Narcolepsy about their school-related issues growing up. They reported a history of falling asleep in class, decreased performance, interpersonal conflicts with teachers, embarrassment due to their symptoms, difficulty making friends, and frequently missing school days. So, what we may have been labeling as behaviorally disturbed children may be really sleepy children! And what we label as unmotivated adolescent behavior may actually be the sleepiness of Narcolepsy!

Narcolepsy in children and adolescents can be associated with:

- Impaired school performance and decreased grades
- Decreased concentration and memory

- Increased discipline troubles at home and school
- Nighttime anxiety or behavioral problems due to insomnia or unrecognized hypnogogic hallucinations
- Children and adolescents may miss a lot of school due to sleepiness and the inability to get up in the morning
- Stress on the family
- Social impairment and struggling to meet/maintain friends
- Bullying in school due to sleepiness, falling asleep in class, and cataplexy
- A possible delay in sexual development due to increased anxiety and avoidance from sleepiness and cataplexy
- Trouble getting up in the morning on their own
- Driving issues
- Low self-esteem
- Avoidance and isolation

It can be associated with "anosmia" or the loss of smell in children. Some may report things to smell funny and not like they used to, "hyposmia." (de Martin Truzzi et al., 2020).

Sudden weight gain and obesity occur in children with Narcolepsy. You can often see weight gain present just as the symptoms of excessive daytime sleepiness develop. Palhano and associates (2018) reported, "The incidence of overweight or obesity ranges from 25% to 74% in patients with Narcolepsy type 1, while precocious puberty is present in 17% of children having narcolepsy with cataplexy. However, the mechanisms involved in the association of Narcolepsy with obesity and precocious puberty have not been fully elucidated yet." Further studies (Plazzi et al., 2018) (Morin, 2020) found "Pediatric narcolepsy is also associated with comorbidities including rapid weight gain, precocious puberty, attention hyperactivity disorder, and increased risk for deficits in social functioning, depression, and anxiety. School performance is also typically impaired, requiring special education services."

Psychiatric and sleep disorders also often co-exist with Narcolepsy in the pediatric and adolescent population. Szakács and associates (2015) studied the psychiatric comorbidity and cognitive profile in children with Narcolepsy. They reported 43% psychiatric comorbidity in children with Narcolepsy, with the following findings:

- ADHD—29%
- Depressive Symptoms—25%
- Major Depressive Disorder—20%
- Generalized Anxiety Disorder—10%
- Oppositional Defiant Disorder—7%
- Pervasive Developmental Disorder NOS—3%
- Eating Disorder NOS—3%

Their cognitive assessment showed average full-scale IQ and perceptual speed results but decreased verbal comprehension and working memory. Those with psychiatric comorbidities did have lower full-scale IQ findings. The psychiatric symptom most frequently found was temper tantrums.

Children with Narcolepsy can also have other sleep disorders like restless legs syndrome, periodic limb movement disorder, and REM sleep behavior disorder. Iron deficiency can also contribute to restless legs symptoms and sleep disruption in pediatric/adolescent patients.

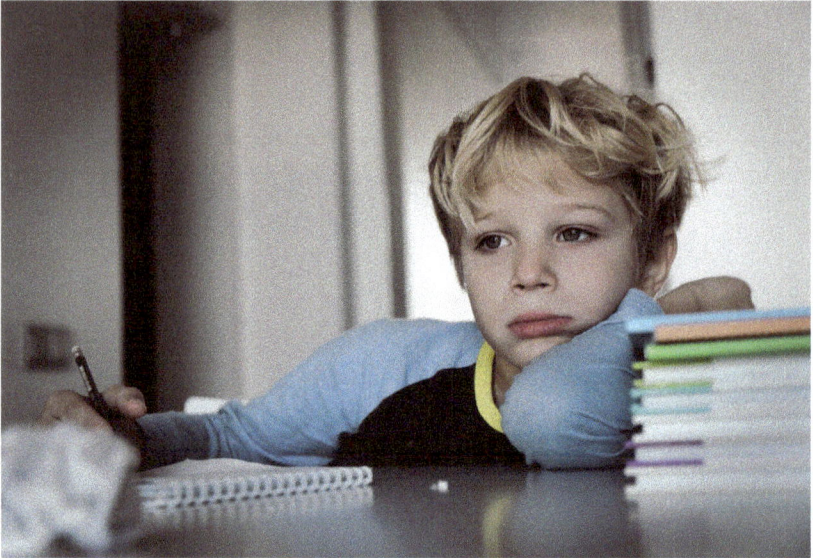

Treatment of Narcolepsy in the Pediatric Population

Supportive psychotherapy, family therapy, and peer support groups can benefit the child or adolescent with Narcolepsy and their family. The Wake Up Narcolepsy group has a support group for parents of people with Narcolepsy. The Narcolepsy Network has a national support group meeting for parents and supporters of people with Narcolepsy. I am sure there are others out there too.

The pharmacological treatment of pediatric Narcolepsy does not have as many FDA-approved options as for adults. Off-label antidepressants are used for cataplexy and various symptoms in the pediatric population but carry a black box warning about suicidal ideation for the pediatric and adolescent populations. Sodium Oxybate is FDA-approved starting at seven years of age for Narcolepsy, and the stimulants methylphenidate and dextroamphetamine are approved for those six and over for ADHD and are often used for Narcolepsy too. Other stimulants and the wake-promoting agents modafinil (Provigil) and armodafinil (Nuvigil) have also been used. Atomoxetine (Strattera), while approved for ADHD over the age of six, has been used for sleepiness and cataplexy in children but is not FDA-approved for those conditions. Other medications are currently seeking pediatric indications with the FDA. Pitolisant (Wakix) recently had significantly improved clinical data in phase three clinical trials in children ages six years and up, and their company is hoping to get FDA approval in pediatric/ adolescent Narcolepsy disorder.

The behavioral recommendations described previously in Chapter 5 of this book are also helpful in the pediatric/adolescent population with some age-adjusted recommendations. In the book *Narcolepsy* (2010), Paruthi and Kotagal include an excellent table on managing children and adolescents with Narcolepsy (Table 6.6), which includes things like using medications for sleepiness and cataplexy, keeping a regular sleep schedule with planned naps, exercise to aid with sleepiness, emotional support, teaching coping skills, sitting in the front of the classroom at school, evaluating for other issues such as depression and precocious puberty, vocational guidance, and supervision when/if they start driving.

Helpful suggestions from Harvard Medical School can be found on their website, such as staying active during class, taking a 15 to 20-minute nap at school and a brief nap after school, remaining active while studying, taking an exercise break, avoiding being sleep-deprived, and keeping a regular sleep schedule.

As mentioned earlier, another important consideration with pediatric Narcolepsy is monitoring for weight gain and precocious puberty with aggressive treatment of both should they be present. If weight gain is significant and snoring is present, evaluation for sleep apnea may be necessary, as sleep apnea does occur in the pediatric population. Laboratory evaluation for other possible contributing factors to weight gain (such as thyroid abnormalities) and iron deficiency, which may contribute to co-existing restless legs syndrome or periodic limb movement disorder, is also indicated.

A book of interest with helpful ideas for various sleep issues in children is *The Rested Child* by W. Chris Winter, MD. Dr. Winter is an internationally known sleep specialist with a unique talent for writing in a very conversational and readable way. Earlier in this book, I recommended his general sleep guide called *The Sleep Solution,* and I think both books are very informative for those living with Narcolepsy and their families.

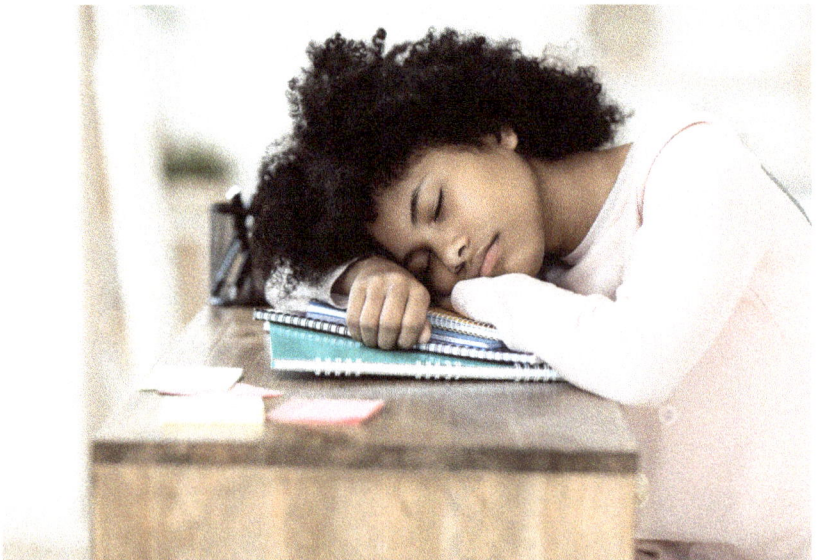

Academic accommodations are always helpful for students with Narcolepsy, and these will be discussed more in Chapter 11. It is essential to know that accommodations should be made throughout school, including college, med school, law school, dental school, etc. While symptoms may change with age, issues may still impair peak performance.

Another exciting development to report is Project Sleep's "Jack & Jill Scholarship" for high school and college students with Narcolepsy planning to go to college/university. Check out their website for more information.

Chapter 7

Sleepy, Worried, and Sad

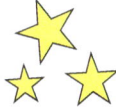

⭐
⭐ ⭐

Depression, Anxiety, and Narcolepsy

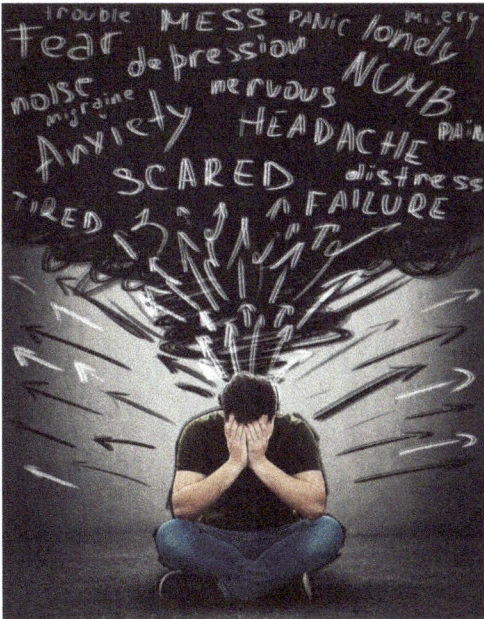

*"You're mourning the loss of what you thought your
life was going to be. Let it go. Things don't always work out how
you plan. That's not necessarily bad. Things have
a way of working out anyway!"*
Dr. Crane from the sitcom Frasier

Psychiatric and other neurologic disorders may share common presentations, and Narcolepsy may be associated with various neuropsychiatric manifestations. BaHammam and associates (2020) reported the complex nature of Narcolepsy, as well as the frequent use of stimulants and anti-cataplectic medications (such as antidepressants) for other disorders, can complicate and delay the diagnosis of Narcolepsy. They reported, "comorbid neuropsychiatric manifestations in patients with Narcolepsy include depression, anxiety, psychosis, rapid eye movement (REM) sleep behavior disorder, and cognitive impairment."

High rates of psychiatric comorbidity and increased psychiatric medication usage were reported with Narcolepsy in the Burden of Narcolepsy Disease (BOND) study by Ruoff and associates (2017). All categories of mental illness were significantly more prevalent, with the highest rates being depression and anxiety. Increased psychiatric medication use was reported with SSRI antidepressants, benzodiazepines, hypnotics, SNRI antidepressants, and tricyclic antidepressants.

A survey of 371 patients (Neikrug and associates 2017), with 65% having Narcolepsy and 34.8% having Idiopathic Hypersomnia, revealed 80% or more reported a sad mood, lost interest, or irritability, and 91% reported trouble with concentration.

Others (Morse and Sanjeev 2018) discussed the association and overlap of Narcolepsy with depression, ADHD, anxiety, schizophrenia, and eating disorders and the overlapping benefit of some pharmacological treatments for these disorders. Comparisons between depression and Narcolepsy revealed both as having sleep difficulties, potential weight changes (increased with Narcolepsy), poor work/school performance, and social isolation.

The Nexus Narcolepsy Registry (Ohayon et al., 2021) study was a longitudinal, web-based registry of real-world experiences of people with Narcolepsy and indicated psychiatric disorders such as depression, anxiety, bipolar disorder, schizophrenia, and ADHD were reported. This study compared the patient's self-reported diagnosis to those confirmed by professional evaluation. Depression was a widespread self-reported misdiagnosis (pediatric onset, 34.2%; adult onset, 29.1%). ADHD was also frequently misdiagnosed, particularly when symptoms presented during childhood, although 9% of pediatric-onset and 11% of adult-onset participants self-reported a correct diagnosis of comorbid ADHD. They reported about a third of patients were correctly diagnosed with depression and about a quarter with anxiety. The significance of this implies we must get the correct diagnosis to ensure adequate treatment and peak performance.

Excessive daytime sleepiness can occur with many physical and psychiatric issues. As found in the Nexus Narcolepsy study, patients with Narcolepsy are often first diagnosed with depression, whether or not it is truly present. Providers may be quick to diagnose depression, especially if the answer is not immediately apparent, for example, in those having Narcolepsy without cataplexy. These disorders are not mutually exclusive, and as stated previously, psychiatric disorders often co-exist.

Psychiatric disorders associated with hypersomnia include bipolar disorder, depression, dysthymia or persistent depressive disorder, premenstrual dysphoric disorder, schizophrenia, and schizoaffective disorder. The hypersomnia of Narcolepsy can appear the same. Dr. Stephen Stahl and I recorded a video on the *Psychiatric Times* website entitled "Psychiatric Comorbidities & Differential Diagnosis in Narcolepsy," which may be helpful.

Narcolepsy and Depression

Patients can have depression before Narcolepsy or as a result of Narcolepsy and the difficulties it causes. The struggle to find the diagnosis and frustration from severe sleepiness and the obstacles it has caused can undoubtedly lead to increased depression. Also, once diagnosed with Narcolepsy, there may be some grief about the diagnosis or anger about the length of time it has taken to find an answer and the missed opportunities. Academic, work, and relationship impairments can lead to depression. The lack of understanding from others can increase depression, anxiety, and isolation. Allow for the sadness. There are no quick fixes, but there are multiple options and resources.

Things to consider when evaluating for depression or anxiety versus Narcolepsy include:

- Is there sleepiness during periods when depression is not present?
- When did the sleepiness start?
- Were they sleepy heads in school?
- Are there other family members who have Narcolepsy or other sleep disorders?

Both depression and Narcolepsy may be present and need to be dealt with. My recommendation is to treat both simultaneously . . . and aggressively! If you wait to find or treat a patient with Narcolepsy without depression, you are missing a lot of Narcolepsy! A provider once told me, "I want to treat the depression first and then wait to see what we are left with concerning the Narcolepsy before we treat it." It would be a shame to leave a patient hanging with many symptoms of Narcolepsy. Back to the metaphor of diabetes, we would not say we want to treat their diabetes before we address their heart disease or hypertension. We would treat all disorders present simultaneously!

Also, sometimes providers have misdiagnosed the cataplexy of Narcolepsy as a seizure disorder, conversion disorder, pseudo seizure, "something psych," or even substance abuse. Cataplexy should at least be in the differential for patients having unusual presentations of muscle weakness or movements.

Narcolepsy and Anxiety

Anxiety disorders are also prevalent in Narcolepsy. Panic attacks are often about the fear of losing control of their body with cataplexy or falling asleep in a public place. Social anxiety is common and is also usually around the fear of falling asleep or having cataplexy in public. Patients who report nocturnal panic-like symptoms may actually be waking with sleep paralysis. Medications such as wake-promoting agents and stimulants can also contribute to anxiety in the Narcolepsy patient.

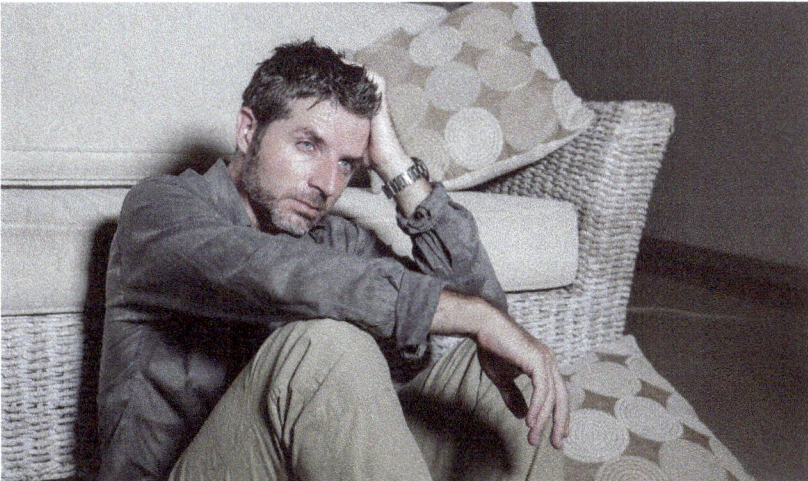

Narcolepsy and Schizophrenia

Comparisons between Narcolepsy and schizophrenia revealed both disorders had associated findings of excessive sleepiness, disrupted sleep, and impaired school/work/cognition issues, which can be associated with other sleep disorders. Distinguishing factors are found between the hallucinations, which are usually visual/multi-modal in Narcolepsy and auditory in Schizophrenia. Hallucinations in Narcolepsy can be complex and multi-sensory. One point to consider with hallucinations is whether they occur only with the transition into or out of sleep (or even with sleep paralysis), indicating Narcolepsy, or are they more persistent throughout the day, which would suggest schizophrenia. Also, those having hypnogogic or hypnopompic hallucinations associated with Narcolepsy are usually aware they are not real. Another rare cause of psychosis in Narcolepsy would be that induced by stimulants. Cataplexy (which is muscle weakness associated with emotion) is found in Narcolepsy, and catatonia (which is a disorder of awareness, lack of responsiveness, abnormal posturing, and confusion that sometimes can be associated with restlessness or agitation) is found in schizophrenia. On rare occasions, patients can have both schizophrenia and Narcolepsy. Dr. Haramandeep Singh and I recorded a case presentation of Schizoaffective Disorder with Narcolepsy, which can be viewed at the *Psychiatric Times* website.

Narcolepsy and ADHD

ADHD is commonly misdiagnosed in pediatric or adolescent patients with Narcolepsy due to the lack of concentration, hyperactivity, or fidgetiness to avoid sleepiness, academic difficulties, and irritability. But these disorders can co-occur. Kim and associates (Kim et al., 2020) published results stating, "The prevalence of ADHD symptoms was >30% in Narcolepsy. Also, the combo of ADHD and Narcolepsy can lead to discouragement and depression."

So, as you can see, there are many co-existing psychiatric and behavioral issues that may be present in the clinical presentation of Narcolepsy. All disorders should be recognized and treated simultaneously to provide the best possible treatment outcome.

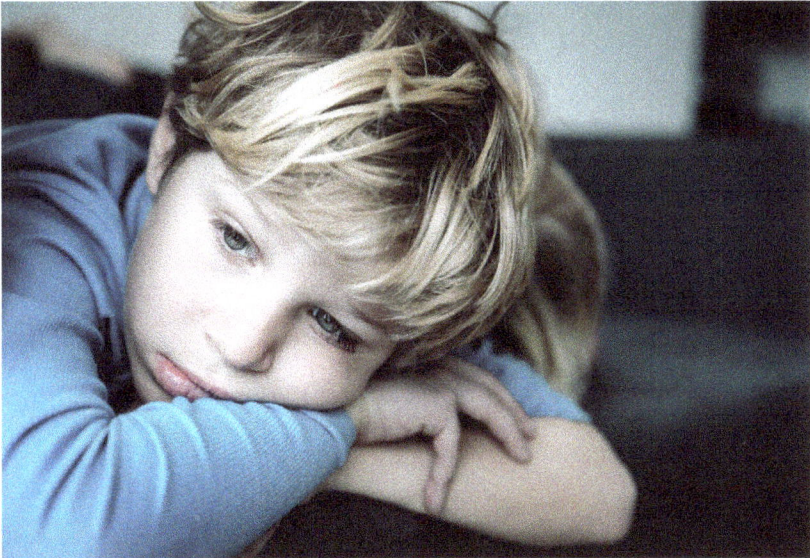

Chapter 8

Narcolepsy Plus One

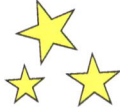

Narcolepsy and Pregnancy

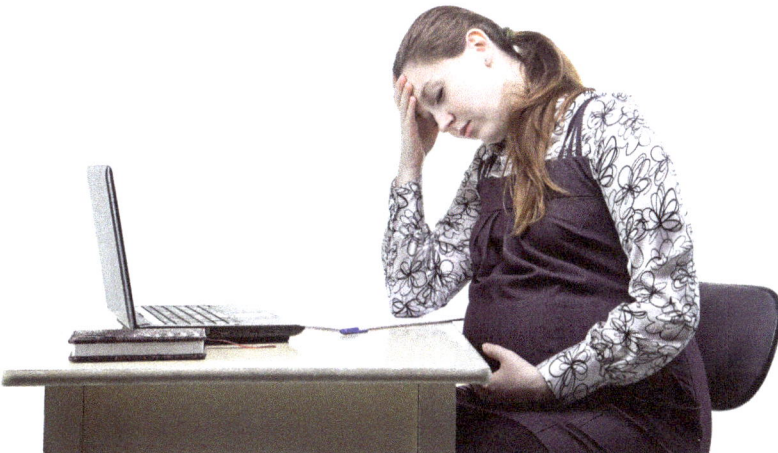

My term for the pregnant Narcolepsy patient:
"Sleepiness Squared! EDS^2"

There's tired, and there is pregnancy tired . . . and then . . . there is the pregnant Narcolepsy tired!

As pregnancy is a time of increased fatigue and sleepiness for women without Narcolepsy, those having excessive daytime sleepiness and Narcolepsy are especially vulnerable during the time of pregnancy. There are so many things to consider about pregnancy when you have Narcolepsy. I would not let this diagnosis keep you from having a child if that is your desire, but serious conversations should occur between you and your partner, your family, and your physician. One must consider the risks or benefits of taking and not taking medications during pregnancy. Suppose your cataplexy or excessive daytime sleepiness is severe when you are not taking medications. In that case, there may be safety issues you may need to consider if you decide not to take medicines during your pregnancy. It could influence your ability to drive, work, and do other activities. FMLA may need to be considered. If you find out you are pregnant and decide to stop meds, then there needs to be a discussion of how to taper and stop the medications.

Abruptly stopping meds can lead to rebound cataplexy and increased sleepiness. Another option to keep in mind would be simplifying the number of medicines you use if you must use meds during pregnancy and using medications that treat both EDS and cataplexy, such as pitolisant (Wakix) or the oxybates (Xyrem/Xywav/Lumryz). Case reports on Narcolepsy medications used during pregnancy are out there, but good studies of intentional use during pregnancy are still lacking. Rare reports of cataplexy during delivery have been reported (Ping et al., 2007) (Ajayi et al., 2012), but delivery is usually without issue.

I have a case I reported on in *The Case Book Of Sleep Medicine*, *3rd Edition* (2019), where I followed a patient with Narcolepsy through two different pregnancies, using sodium oxybate (Xyrem) during both pregnancies. The patient had normal deliveries on both occasions, and both babies had average Apgar scores at one minute and five minutes. There were no developmental issues afterward. My patient told me during her second pregnancy, even while on medications, "I have never been more tired in my life."

Of course, she had a young child at home, was pregnant, and had Narcolepsy. This case, I think, brings up an interesting point in that you must consider the risks/benefits of treatment of Narcolepsy during pregnancy of the unborn child and the Mother, but also other children that may be at home, work responsibilities, academic advancements, couples' issues/intimacy, driving safety, and a host of other factors when deciding on treatment during pregnancy.

My patient stopped her sodium oxybate after her second delivery due to her nighttime demands with both children. Still, in severely sleepy people with extreme Narcolepsy, one option would be to take medicine and have someone else be in charge of the nighttime feedings and demands of the baby, such as the partner, grandmother, hired babysitter, etc.

Most drugs may not be toxic, but we do not have a lot of studies on them. Some patients on treatments for Narcolepsy may have had children with some difficulties that may or may not be related to the meds. Using medications may depend on the severity of the illness, as safety issues are of concern. Thorpy and associates (Thorpy et al., 2013) (Thorpy, 2016b) reported that "the perceived risks of Narcolepsy medication during pregnancy to the mother and the fetus usually are overestimated, as the risk for teratogenic effects from Narcolepsy medications in therapeutic doses is essentially nonexistent. However, the potential for rare complications during pregnancy and congenital abnormalities cannot be excluded. Most Narcolepsy patients have vaginal delivery without complications. In rare cases patients had cataplexy that interfered with delivery, but if a caesarian is required, there appears to be no increased anesthetic or surgical risks." The Hypersomnia Foundation has a "Pregnancy Risk Profiles of Medications" (under their resources tab reviewing meds during pregnancy) that is a good review source.

There are four primary areas for females to consider concerning Narcolepsy and pregnancy:

1) Narcolepsy and birth control: Provigil (modafinil), Nuvigil (armodafinil), and Wakix (pitolisant) can decrease the effectiveness of oral contraceptive pills. They can still be used with the appropriate alternative birth control techniques. The alternative methods would need to be used for three weeks after discontinuing some of these meds. Sunosi (solriameftol) may be a safer alternative concerning effective birth control pill use and fertility.

2) Using meds if you do get pregnant throughout the pregnancy: The Hypersomnia Foundation review of "Pregnancy Risk Profiles of Medications" under their "Parenthood & Pregnancy" resource is highly informative. I strongly suggest you review it and discuss options with your OB/GYN or high-risk pregnancy OB physician.

3) Delivery considerations: There have been rare reports of cataplexy with delivery, as mentioned above, but generally, delivery is without complications except for the fatigue and sleepiness that may be present with prolonged labor.

4) Options after delivery if you are breastfeeding: Fatigue, sleepiness, sleep deprivation due to hormonal fluctuations, disrupted nocturnal sleep, and increased demands of caring for the baby should all be considered when deciding to breastfeed when you have Narcolepsy. Your available help at night can weigh into the decision as well. If you are going to breastfeed and decide to take medications, try to do it just before you take any medicine (so the lowest levels of meds would be in your system) and pump milk to allow feedings when you are incredibly sleepy or napping and when others care for the child. Some Mothers report they fall asleep breastfeeding, which can occur even in those without Narcolepsy. However, always try breastfeeding with a supportive pillow under the baby in a safe environment and

with someone else present when possible. If necessary, you may need to breastfeed and pump milk right afterward, and then right after breastfeeding, you can take a short-acting stimulant. You can use the pumped milk for the next feeding. Another option would be using donor milk.

Additionally, other things to consider as contributing to sleepiness during pregnancy besides just Narcolepsy would include:

Obstructive sleep apnea (OSA): There is an increased risk of OSA during pregnancy with increased weight and sinus congestion. This may develop for the first time or increase in severity during pregnancy. A home sleep study or in-lab study is indicated with snoring or increased sleepiness. CPAP may need to be considered. Vicks VapoRub for nasal congestion and over-the-nose snore guards are other options. Elevating the head of the bed and avoiding sleeping on the back may also be helpful.

Restless Legs Syndrome (RLS): Restless Legs Syndrome is an uncomfortable feeling in the legs leading to the desire to move, stretch, and rub the legs. It can also occur in the arms. RLS is more prevalent during pregnancy, especially in the 3rd trimester. Prenatal vitamins with their iron and magnesium may be helpful for these symptoms, as can Epsom salt soaks or rubbing magnesium oil on the legs, but their use must be cleared first before use by your OB/GYN.

Other medical disorders: Other disorders that could be contributing to excessive daytime sleepiness and fatigue include anemia, glucose abnormalities, hypothyroidism, and nutritional insufficiencies. Your physician can do lab work to check for these.

Depression and anxiety: Anxiety about delivery and demands after the baby is born, as well as post-partum depression with decreased energy and low motivation, may contribute to fatigue and sleepiness.

Therapy and support groups can be beneficial during this time. At times, medications may be necessary. Transcranial Magnetic Stimulation (TMS) may be used during pregnancy and when breastfeeding for resistant depression without danger to the child.

Increased progesterone: Increased progesterone during the 1st trimester of pregnancy can lead to increased drowsiness.

Heartburn or gastroesophageal reflux: Increased abdominal size pushing up on the diaphragm leads to increased gastroesophageal reflux, which disrupts sleep. Avoiding heavy meals before bedtime, sleeping with your head elevated, and avoiding spicy foods are other helpful interventions. Medications may be necessary.

Pain and edema: Changing body size and proportions in the pregnant patient can lead to increased pain and discomfort. Supportive positioning of body pillows may be helpful. Side sleeping with the knees bent may be beneficial. A hot bath before bedtime may help to relax muscles and promote overall relaxation. Light stretching or yoga may relieve tired muscles. A partner massage can be helpful. Elevation of your feet and legs before bedtime may help to decrease edema. Avoid salt and other foods promoting edema. Try foot rubs and soaks. Sleeping with your head elevated can also be helpful. Ensuring the temperature of the room is not too hot can increase comfort.

Fetal movements: You may notice if certain foods or drinks increase your baby's movements at night. Rubbing your belly, soft music, singing to your baby, and being calm about it could even lead to increased comfort, reassurance, and habits for the baby.

Other possibilities: Other potential issues include breast tenderness, morning sickness, and frequent bathroom visits.

Cataplexy during pregnancy and delivery may also be increased due to increased emotion, laughter, joy, surprise, etc. Awareness of this and considering safety issues during and after the pregnancy is necessary. If significant cataplexy is present, medications may be the safest option for both the baby and the Mother.

Recent studies on the association of other medical issues during pregnancy in Narcoleptic patients have been reported, such as that by Wilson and associates (2022), which found "significant positive associations between Narcolepsy and the following risk factors and pregnancy-related conditions: maternal obesity, anemia, pre-pregnancy hypertension and diabetes, and gestational hypertension." These findings suggest close supervision for other disorders is warranted during pregnancy. The Wilson study and another by Calvo-Ferrandiz and Peraita-Adrados (2018) indicated no increased rate of preterm labor or cesarean sections with Narcolepsy.

Another topic I must mention is co-sleeping with your baby if you have Narcolepsy. It would, in my opinion, be much better to have a bassinet in the room or a carry bassinet in the bed, a baby bed, or have the baby in the baby room with a monitor rather than co-sleeping with a baby in the bed when we suspect you will be very sleepy and sleep deprived. You can reconsider this option as the baby gets bigger and you are less tired.

Get your support lined up. Ask for help. Identify your support team and have them available at various times of the day or night, especially at first. Make a schedule for everyone. Get someone helping at night. Schedule your naps. Sleep when you can, and have others help with household responsibilities and the baby. Limit visitors to arrive only during **your** awake periods. Schedule alone time with your partner as well. Rest and recharge!

And don't forget, Fathers and other partners with Narcolepsy may become incredibly tired from the sleep deprivation of being a new parent and worry about their partner during pregnancy and delivery. The family may not appreciate the significance of their Narcolepsy symptoms for the spouse or partner. Don't forget about "Dear Old Dad" or the other pregnancy partners. They may have Narcolepsy too!

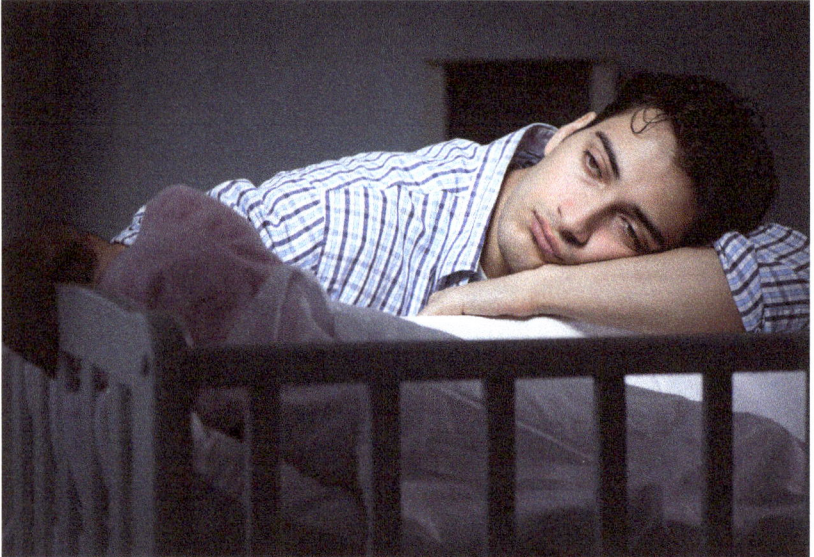

My final suggestion is to join the Wake Up Narcolepsy Support Group "Pregnancy & Parenting With Narcolepsy," or another peer support group focused on this issue. Also, the Project Sleep group has a "Pregnancy & Narcolepsy Toolkit" and a "Pregnancy & Narcolepsy" Podcast. Their toolkit lists the specific potential side effects of medications for Narcolepsy during pregnancy and tips to use throughout pregnancy and after the baby arrives.

Narcolepsy and Pregnancy Patient Comments

"I'm a walking ZOMBIE, and I think I'm going to be like that for a while without my medications!"
Anonymous patient

"I'm just MISERABLE without my medicine!"
A patient, at 35 weeks pregnant and not taking meds

"You know you're a Mom when your fantasies are about sleeping."
Anonymous on the internet

"People who say they sleep like a baby usually don't have one."
Leo J. Burke

"I get really sleepy and sometimes fall asleep while breastfeeding."
Anonymous patient.

Chapter 9

"We Are Family"

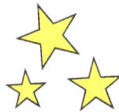

Narcolepsy and Your Family

"Everyone tells you what's good for you. They don't want you to find your own answers.

They want you to believe theirs."

Dan Millman, Way of the Peaceful Warrior

Your family . . . give them time. You don't understand this disorder completely, and they may still be in denial. Let's give them resources. Let's invite them to visit Project Sleep, Wake Up Narcolepsy, and the Narcolepsy Network. Let's give them Julie Flygare's book, *Wide Awake and Dreaming*. Let's provide them with this book. Let's share some websites and a couple of TED Talks. You ask them not to judge you, so don't judge them—show them the way, gently. They don't want you to be ill. They want you to be okay and hope your illness is not so severe. They feel helpless too. In trying to help, they may give many suggestions, some of which may be helpful and others that may feel insulting. Let's give them grace and show them the path to understanding. It's a struggle. You don't understand; they don't understand.

A supportive family member or friend can make all the difference. One of my patients described the difference she noticed when she moved closer to her Father and Stepmother, who understood her disorder and were very supportive, as opposed to living near her Mother, where she felt constantly criticized. She stated, "I seem to be mostly triggered by negative emotions." She reported increased sleepiness and cataplexy when she had a conflict with her Mother. She felt more acceptance and help from her Father and Stepmother daily. Her symptoms improved, and other issues stabilized. She felt more in control. She was more accepting of the illness and herself. She described it as "Now it is Jennifer and Narcolepsy, not Narcolepsy and Jennifer . . . I took my life back!"

Family members need to talk about their frustrations about this disorder too; although one person has the disease, the family, their system, and their plans and activities are affected. They need to feel heard and appreciated too. You may feel like a burden, frustrated, and alone, but in another line from Julie Flygare's book, "You are not a burden. You HAVE a burden, which by definition is too heavy to carry on your own."

Create your team—family members, friends, teachers, co-workers, and support groups. Consider making it your mission to share accurate information with others. We need to educate teachers more about the specifics of this disorder. Teachers can help, especially with younger kids. They can notice the sleepiness in school, the lack of participation, and the incomplete work.

Does anyone else in your family have a sleep disorder or have been told they are a "sleepy head"? As I mentioned earlier in the book, I had a patient whose Father died in a head-on MVA, and he had about five accidents before his death. He was not diagnosed with Narcolepsy, but you certainly would wonder. Do you have family members with frequent accidents? Your family members may realize others in the family have similar symptoms. Narcolepsy can run in the family, especially with the first-degree relatives who may have a 10–40x increased risk of Narcolepsy, although the overall general risk is still low. There is an increased risk of Narcolepsy and other neurologic disorders in families. I once had two sisters, both with myotonic dystrophy and both with Narcolepsy. I have several Mother/daughter families with Narcolepsy. I have one family with three family members severely affected by Narcolepsy. So, look around.

And remember, having someone in the family (or friend circle) with Narcolepsy definitely affects everyone!

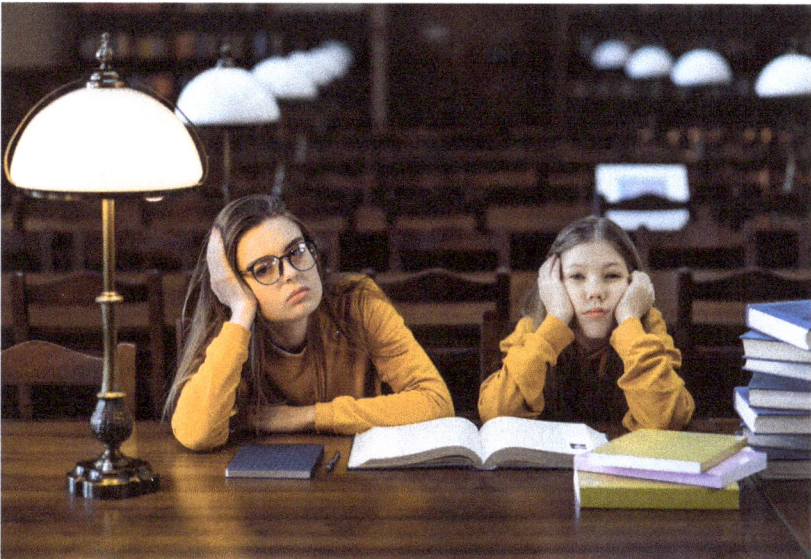

Common effects of Narcolepsy on the patient and their inner circle of support include:

- Rescheduling activities due to sleepiness or cataplexy
- Insomnia is disruptive at night for others
- Missed activities at school, family functions, and after-school activities
- Increased accidents
- Increased absence from work/school
- Increased need for short-term disability or even total disability
- Job loss
- Early retirement
- Relationship issues/divorce

Suggestions for Friends and Family Members of the Person with Narcolepsy

You must seek and learn about this disorder as a family member. It can bring you much closer; if you don't, you risk increased conflict due to uncertainty. Ask your loved one what they need; don't just tell them what you think they need to do. What they need will change day to day as this disease is variable. Look at the resources available. Let them know you are ready to learn. Sometimes, just being available to listen is all you need to do. As it is said, "Be present—not perfect."

"When a chronically ill person says, 'I'm tired,' and you say, 'Yeah, me too, I got five hours of sleep last night,' please understand that you and that person are not talking about the same kind of tiredness." This is from the Chronic Pain Princess from Tumblr about Lupus—but applies to Narcolepsy too. It is not helpful to say, "I know what you mean. I have not slept well." **It is estimated that**

non-narcoleptic individuals must go up to 48—72 hours without sleep at all to attain the same degree of sleepiness a Narcolepsy patient faces every day. That comparison is like comparing a river to the ocean, with the vast degree of sleepiness knocking down the Narcolepsy patient at times like the crashing of the ocean waves.

> *"Don't rush to fix things. Or give advice. Sometimes, people just need to vent. And to feel heard."*
>
> *Author Diane Tarantini, on her Facebook page*

The worst thing you can do to someone with an illness is to make them feel like they need to prove how sick they are or dismiss their symptoms. If you have a friend or family member with Narcolepsy, accept them where they are. Help them devise a plan to make it better. Make accommodations. Schedule activities at their most alert times of the day. Ask them how you can be supportive. Maybe they need you to listen. Perhaps they need you to pick up the kids or a few groceries. Maybe they just need a hug. Seek out knowledge about Narcolepsy. Show them you are interested and trying. Join a support group.

> *"Sometimes all they really need is a hand to hold, an ear to listen, and a heart to understand them."*
>
> *Zig Ziglar*

Like AA for alcoholics and Al-Anon for the families of alcoholics, we have Narcolepsy support groups for patients and others for the families of Narcolepsy patients. I can't say enough about the importance of peer support in treating Narcolepsy! Having others who understand you and your daily struggles is absolutely priceless. There are local support groups in some areas and support groups online with the Narcolepsy Network and Wake Up Narcolepsy for both patients and their support teams. The Narcolepsy Network has a "National Support Group Meeting for People with Narcolepsy" and a "National Support Group Meeting for Parents/Supporters of People with Narcolepsy." The Wake Up Narcolepsy website has several groups such as "Living with Narcolepsy," "Living with Narcolepsy—Canada," "Living with Narcolepsy—LGBTQIA+," "College & Careers with Narcolepsy," and "Pregnancy and Parenting with Narcolepsy." Imagine being in a room (even virtually) with others who understand you and the effects of Narcolepsy! The Project Sleep website has a "Rising Voices" program where patients share their stories about living with Narcolepsy. These are very interesting. These videos may be beneficial for friends and family members to learn more about Narcolepsy. Look for resources. I am sure there are others. Be a part of the team.

Additionally, I always feel like individual and couples/family therapy are helpful for those with significant Narcolepsy, just as we would recommend it in those with severe breast cancer, leukemia, depression, anxiety, patients on dialysis, or any other severe chronic illness. Find a good local therapist.

"There is a story behind every person.
There is a reason why they are.

Think about that and respect them for who they are."

marcandangel

Let's Talk About Sex!

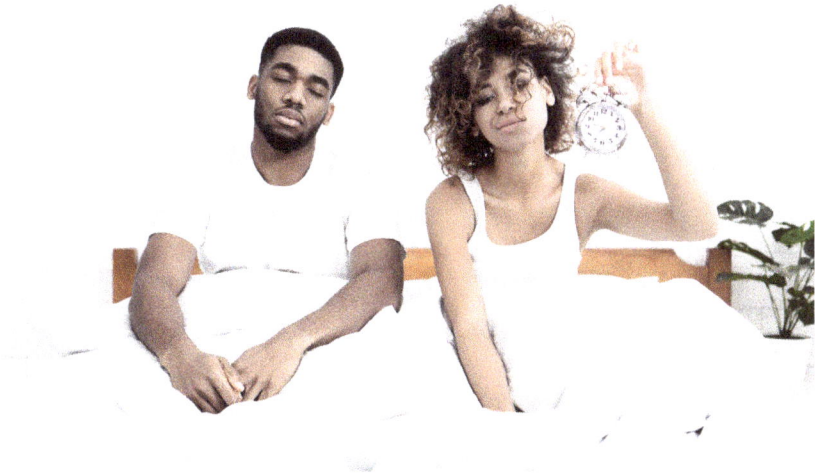

An article by Davidson and associates (2022) entitled "The impact of Narcolepsy on social relationships in young adults" reported that 81% of the patients surveyed felt Narcolepsy impacted their sex life. Still, only a few (9.8%) felt their providers asked about their sex lives, and (69%) reported their clinician asked about the social impact of their disorder. Of the 238 patients questioned, 32% experienced cataplexy during sex, and 53% indicated they had fallen asleep during sex. So, the lesson here is that for the providers reading this book, we need to ask about how Narcolepsy interferes with our patient's sex life and social relationships. For the people with Narcolepsy reading this book, please bring these issues up with your providers! Please don't wait for them to ask.

In Julie Flygare's book, she gave terrific descriptions of the effect Narcolepsy had on her sex life. On p.32, she stated, "Immediately after this sexual sensation, my head and neck flopped backward against the bed, in a harsh whip-lashing motion." On p.33, she reported, "Being sexually aroused left me limp as a ragdoll." Not everyone has this experience with sexual activity, as not everyone has cataplexy with anger or even laughter. But it can occur, and you should monitor for these symptoms. An intersting report on "orgasmolepsy" in Narcolepsy with response to pitolisant was described by Pellittere et al. 2020 (Pellitteri et al., 2020).

Severe sleepiness can result in decreased libido. Acute sleep deprivation can lead to hypersexuality. One can have sexual arousal-induced cataplexy, and I have even heard of one patient who could not reach orgasm at all due to this situation. Antidepressants may decrease libido and delay orgasm. Impotence can be due to antidepressant use in the Narcoleptic patient or due to cataplexy. Changing to a different antidepressant may be helpful. Viagra or Cialis may be beneficial. Patients with Narcolepsy can fall asleep before sex even starts.

So, what are the options here? First, plan a sexual activity to avoid the periods of your most extreme sleepiness. Have sex during the day when you are most alert and not at the end of the day when you are sleepiest. Leave the lights on. Have sex somewhere other than the bed where you associate going to sleep (like the guest room or other rooms in your house). Look at your music choices during romantic encounters. Consider alerting meds before sex or plan sex after your wake-promoting agents have had time to kick in. Take a nap before your usual time of sex. Help your partner understand. Let your partner help you find a time of day or situation that works best for you and make the necessary environmental adjustments. It can be a fun part of anticipating sexual activity between partners. Of course, there are other forms of intimacy, but do not forget the importance of sex in your relationship. And once again, "a Nappetizer" briefly before sex may help considerably during sex. Relax about it and enjoy!

"The simple act of listening to someone and making them feel as if they have truly been heard is a most treasured gift."

L.A. Villafane

Chapter 10

Finding Help

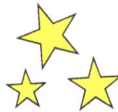

Narcolepsy Resources

"In some cases, we learn more by looking for the answer to a question and not finding it than we do from learning the answer itself."
Lloyd Alexander, The Book of Three

Discovering and learning about this disorder is an essential journey for the patient with Narcolepsy. Finding as many resources and support systems as possible can affect this disorder's day-to-day outcome. The following organizations and resources are just some of the many that I have found helpful. Spend some time reviewing and finding out what works best for you. You should always check your sources, as not everything you see online is always accurate, but you can find plenty of helpful hints. This list is growing daily, so research and update your resources regularly!

- Narcolepsy Network
- Project Sleep
- Wake Up Narcolepsy
- Hypersomniafoundation.org
- Narcolepsy Link
- National Organization for Rare Disorders (NORD)
- Support Groups

There are some interesting and insightful lectures on the internet and social media posted by providers. For example, *NeurologyLive. com* includes various Narcolepsy videos filmed over the years. Search the *Psychiatric Times* website for articles and videos about Narcolepsy. Harvard and Stanford have Narcolepsy tips on their websites, as do other major institutions. The American Academy of Sleep Medicine also has Narcolepsy resources listed. The websites that follow contain a wealth of information about sleep and are well worth a look:

- Sleep Unplugged with Dr. Chris Winter on Apple Podcasts and YouTube
- Narcolepsy UK
- Faces of Narcolepsy (Families and Children Experiencing Symptoms of Narcolepsy)
- Catnap Narcolepsy registry
- @remrunner—Julie Flygare on Twitter
- Women of Narcolepsy
- Rising Voices of Narcolepsy
- Project Sleep Podcasts
- www.Day4NAPS.org
- pwn4pwn.org (People with Narcolepsy for People with Narcolepsy.org)
- CoRDS (Coordination of Rare Diseases at Stanford Research)
- The individual websites for Xyrem/Xywav/Lumryz, Wakix, Sunosi, Provigil, and Nuvigil

YouTube has many videos about Narcolepsy, as mentioned earlier; here are a few more:

- Narcolepsy (NORD)— causes, symptoms, diagnosis, treatment, pathology
- Narcoleptic Dog
- James, the Narcoleptic tree cutter
- Dogs who lost the fight against sleep
- CATAPLEXY ATTACK
- The Narcoleptic Mom
- The nap mistress
- What is Narcolepsy
- Living with Narcolepsy
- Cataplexy videos

An article by Franceschini and associates (2021) provides an international list of Narcolepsy associations across the globe:

- Austria: www.narkolepsie.at
- Belgium: www.narcolepsie-cataplexie.be
- Denmark: www.dansknarkolepsiforening.dk
- France: www.anc-narcolepsie.com
- Germany: http://www.dng-ev.de/
- Ireland: http://soundireland.ie/
- Netherlands: www.narcolepsie.nl
- Norway: http://www.sovnforeningen.no/
- Poland: http://www.narkolepsja.pl/
- Spain: http://www.narcolepsia.org/
- Sweden: http://www.narkolepsiforeningen.se/
- Switzerland: https://www.snane.ch/
- UK: www.narcolepsy.org.uk
- USA: NORD (National Organization for Rare Disorders): https://rarediseases.org/rare-diseases/narcolepsy/
- USA: Wake up Narcolepsy: https://www.wakeupnarcolepsy.org/

- USA: Narcolepsy Network: www.narcolepsynetwork.org
- USA: Project Sleep: https://project-sleep.com/

The information above is only a limited amount of the available websites and educational resources on Narcolepsy. Seek out information, especially regarding your specific situation or co-existing disorders with Narcolepsy. Go to the American Academy of Sleep Medicine website, visit the drug company websites for each of the Narcolepsy medications described in this book, visit the National Sleep Foundation, and search for podcasts. Arm yourself with as much information as possible.

Chapter 11

Developing a Game Plan

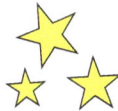

Accommodations for Those with Narcolepsy

*"Sometimes the questions are complicated, and the
answers are simple."*
Dr. Seuss

Sleep. Take a nap when you must! Protect your sleep. Keep your sleep schedule regular. Schedule planned naps. Find what works for you. What works for you now may not always work for you. You change, your Narcolepsy changes, treatment options change, resources change, and your friends/family and social support change. Periodically, you need to re-evaluate. Ask yourself and your provider, "Am I on the best medications I can be on at this moment?" Sometimes, trying a different combination of medicines or even changing the timing of your current medications can be helpful. Are there more resources out there? Are there things you are doing that are no longer working? Are you having more trouble at a specific time of the day (morning versus afternoon versus evening)? Do you need to update your tribe of people? Do you once again need to look at your schedule, responsibilities, and sleep hygiene? Have you changed any medicines, even over-the-counter medications, or supplements, which could increase your sleepiness or other symptoms? Have you had any labs within the last year? Look for accommodations at school, work, and home environments, such as a resting space and place for scheduled naps. Take inventory and step up your treatment plan. Educate those around you.

Ask for help!

Look for resources!

Academic Accommodations for Narcolepsy

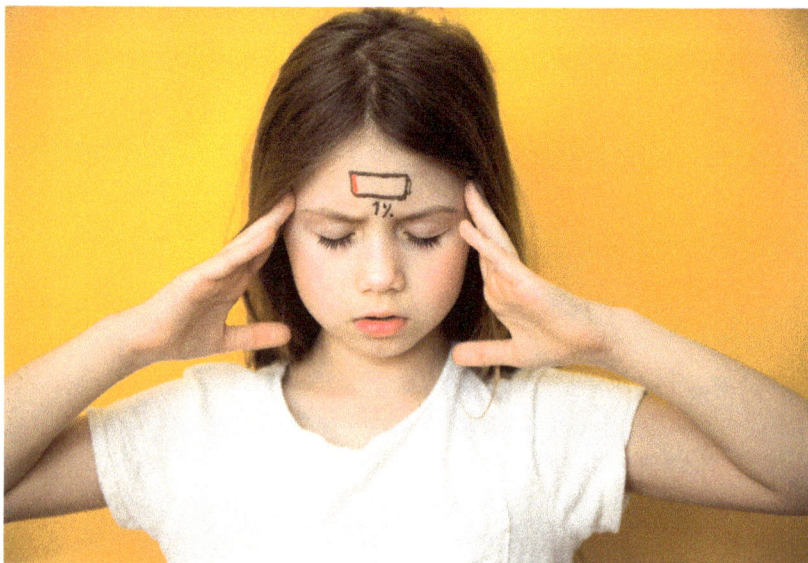

Dealing with school while having Narcolepsy can present multiple obstacles, but assistance is available. Talk to the school officials. Investigate exam conditions so that the stress of the exam does not increase your cataplexy or excessive daytime sleepiness. Look for note-takers or recorders. Sit in the front of the room to avoid distraction or possibly near the door in case you need to leave due to the sedation or impending cataplexy. Find a buddy in class who can assist if necessary or share notes should you have to leave. Find a safe napping space should you need to rejuvenate. Splash water on your face, do some brief exercises, have a treat, or take a quick walk to help alert yourself. Below are some specifics I feel may be helpful that I found at the leading Narcolepsy sites:

Project Sleep
- Podcast "Navigating School with Narcolepsy"
- Jack and Julie Narcolepsy Scholarship
- Can a student with a sleep disorder receive disability accommodations in school?

Wake Up Narcolepsy
- The Student with Narcolepsy and the Education System
- Narcolepsy Accommodations: School & Work
- Brown Bag Webinar: Accommodations For School & Work
- Support Group: College and Careers with Narcolepsy

Narcolepsy Network
- Classroom Accommodations brochure
- 10 Things Educators Should Know
- Narcolepsy in the Classroom Brochure
- SAT and ACT accommodations for students with Narcolepsy
- Sample letter to a high school teacher about a 504 Plan for Education
- Sample letter to a teacher about Narcolepsy

- Example 504 Plan from a student recently diagnosed with Narcolepsy
- Example 504 Plan for a student with Narcolepsy
- Scholarship opportunities for students with disabilities in the US
- Preparing for postsecondary education

Another example of academic interventions with sleep is the **Wake Up and Learn** education program, which is a school-based education and assessment program in Pennsylvania used to improve overall mental, physical, and emotional health and encourages students, parents, and educators to adopt healthy sleep patterns. This was initiated by Dr. Anne Marie Morse and the Janet Weis Children's Hospital at Geisinger Health. They provided sleep education and free sleep assessments to students. A model of this program could certainly be adopted elsewhere to increase the focus of sleep in academic settings.

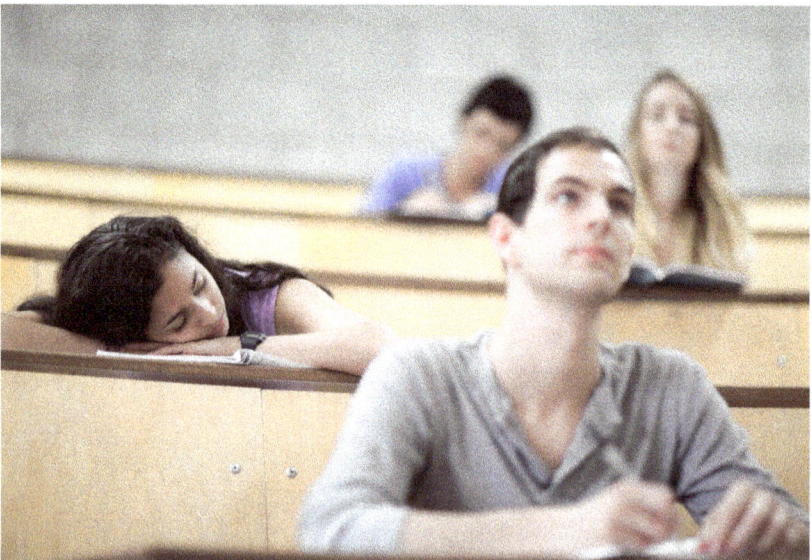

Occupational Accommodations

Working with Narcolepsy, especially if you spend long hours sitting at your desk looking at a computer, can be exhausting and contribute to excessive daytime sleepiness. Keep your workstation and computer files well organized. Give yourself brief breaks. Stand up, stretch, walk, do some quick exercises, grab water or caffeine, or take a power nap if possible. Talk with your employer about the possibility of breaking your lunch break into two brief napping breaks instead of a longer lunch break.

Narcolepsy is a diagnosis covered by the Americans with Disabilities Act, requiring reasonable accommodations, and preventing discrimination for this disorder. The nature of the job, the safety of others, and where you work may influence what would be considered appropriate. As such, you may be able to clock out for one or two brief naps as long as the required workload is completed within a designated time period, and it does not endanger others. This diagnosis would need to be reviewed with your employer to see what options are available. Some employment opportunities would not be ideal for the patient with significant Narcolepsy. As I understand it now, Narcolepsy itself is not usually an approved disorder for Social Security benefits; however, if it affects your ability to work, you may qualify for some benefits. And occasionally, I have had a patient approved for disability. Below are some specific resources available for your review:

Project Sleep
- Narcolepsy at Work
- Nurses with Narcolepsy
- Doctors with Narcolepsy

Wake Up Narcolepsy
- Narcolepsy Accommodations: School & Work brochure
- College and Careers with Narcolepsy support group

Narcolepsy Network
- Job Accommodations Network
- Staying Employed with a Sleep Disorder
- Entrepreneurship and Narcolepsy
- Narcolepsy and Employment: What Are Your Rights?
- Working with Narcolepsy roundtable discussion
- Lime Connect, which connects people with disabilities to employers
- US Equal Employment Opportunity Commission (EEOC), Disability Discrimination

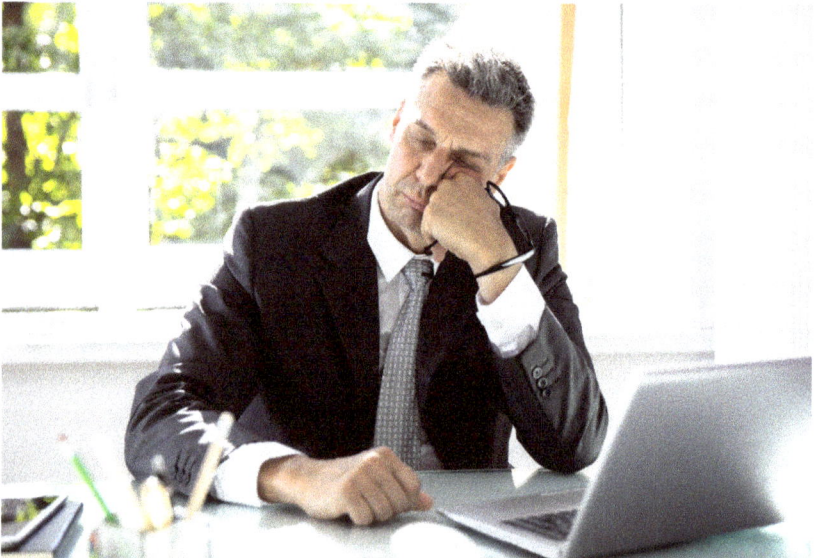

Chapter 12

You Are Not Alone

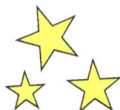

Narcolepsy Is More Common Than You Think

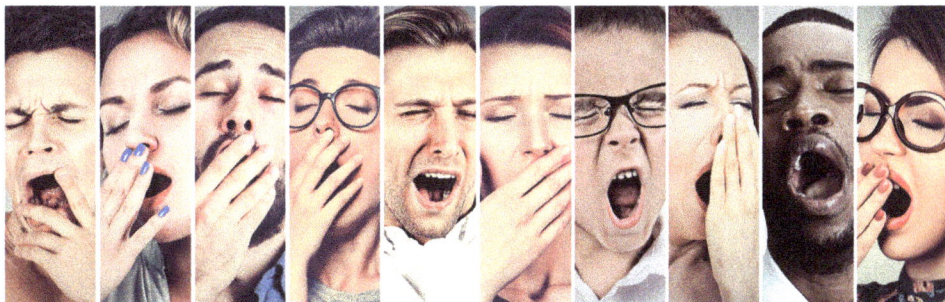

"You're not unreliable—your health is."
@theintuitives

This quote is seen in multiple places online regarding various disorders, emphasizing its importance. The most important person with Narcolepsy is you! Plenty of people with this disorder have lived healthy and productive lives. You can too! There are many famous people with Narcolepsy, and I will list some here to show you that even though Narcolepsy is a disabling disorder, and you will probably need medications and accommodations, the sky is the limit!

In this chapter, I'm also sharing some of the many comments describing the symptoms of Narcolepsy that I have collected over the years from my patients, articles/books I have read, lectures, videos, social media, and years of being interested in this disorder. The symptoms are real, can be variable, can seem strange, may be unusual, and you may not have appreciated that the signs were even a part of your Narcolepsy.

As I said in the Introduction, my patients have taught me so much over the years about this disorder, and their strength and resiliency are inspiring. I wish this for you. I can't say their names, but they are the heroes in this book. Sometimes, I have heard almost the exact same comment from different patients as their symptoms are so similar. I hope as you read the following statements, you realize you fit in. That others feel the same way as you.

Be inspired. You are not alone!

Famous People Reported to Have Narcolepsy

These are listed in various places on the internet, and I have no personal confirmation of their diagnosis.

Late-night comedian Jimmy Kimmel

British Prime Minister Winston Churchill

Baseball player Hank Aaron

Musician Kurt Cobain from the musical group Nirvana

Inventor Thomas Edison

Actress Natassa Kinski

Comedian Lenny Bruce

Author Teresa Nielson Hayden

Activist Harriet Tubman (the female who rescued many enslaved people and suffered Narcolepsy and epilepsy secondary to a head injury)

Educator Louis Braille, the man who invented braille to help people who are blind learn to read

NFL player Josh Andrews

English football goalkeeper Aaron Adam Flahavan

French professional bicycle racer Franck Bouyer, who was disqualified from competing because his Narcolepsy medication was considered a performance-enhancing drug (Modafinil)

British actor Arthur Lowe

Drummer Gabe Barham from the band Sleeping with Sirens

American drag performer Jinkx Monsoon, previously seen on *RuPaul's Drag Race*

Kevin Cadogan from the band Third Eye Blind

Jazz musician Paul Gonsalves

Deputy White House Chief of Staff to Bill Clinton, Harold Ickes

Molecular geneticist, molecular engineer, and chemist from Harvard, George M. Church

Pro golfer on LPGA Nicole Jeray

Author Harriet Scott Chessman, the author of the book *The Beauty of Ordinary Things*

French Film director Henri-Georges Clouzot

Project Sleep's "Doctors with Narcolepsy" and "Nurses with Narcolepsy"

So, look at the list above. These are only a few I know of. Focus on the different jobs and accomplishments. The possibilities are limitless for you too!

TV Shows That Feature Narcolepsy

Several *Seinfeld* episodes discuss Narcolepsy, including when Jerry dates a girl who falls asleep every time Jerry wants to have sex with her; George pretends to have Narcolepsy; and Kramer ends up developing Narcolepsy after taking an off-label Narcolepsy medication for blood pressure.

In *The Simpsons* episode #575, "Every Man's Dream," Homer is diagnosed with Narcolepsy.

The British sitcom *Mr. Bean* showed an example of falling asleep on a rollercoaster in the episode "Mr. Bean Rides the Big One."

Perception TV show which describes sleep paralysis, hypnogogic hallucinations, slurred words, and sleepiness in Season 2, Episode 2, "Alienation"

The Disney Plus series *The Mysterious Benedict Society*, in which Mr. Benedict has Type 1 Narcolepsy, has cataplexy with laughing, and will immediately fall asleep.

In an episode of the sitcom *Frasier*, Niles is thought to have Narcolepsy after his divorce.

Movies That Feature Narcolepsy

Ode to Joy: Jason Winer (2019)

Deuce Bigalow: Male Gigolo: Mike Mitchell (1999)

My Own Private Idaho: Gus Van Sant (1991)

Narco: Tristan Aurojet, Gilles Lellouche (2004)

I Am a Red Man: Thiru (2014)

The Most Beautiful Day: Florian David Fitz (2016)

Venus and Lulu: Daniel Losset (1991)

Moulin Rouge: Baz Luhrmann (2001)

Nobody, Nobody But Juan: Enrico "Eric" Quizon (2009)

Drowsiness: Magdalena Piekorz (2008)

Dead Time: Joko Anwar (2007)

The Three Trials: Randy Grief (2006)

Rat Race: Jerry Zucker (2001)

Hello Again – A Wedding A Day: Maggie Peren (2020)

Very Happy Alexander: Robert Yves (1968)

The Narcoleptic: Eric H. Sheffield (2021)

Naan Sigappu Manithan: Thiru (2014)

Any Minute Now: Peter Goddard (2013)

The Secret Adventures of Gustave Klopp: Tristan Aurouet, Gilles Lellouche (2004)

Centimeters: Ramon Salazar (2005)

An Interesting Article with Descriptions of Narcolepsy

I reviewed a fascinating article, "Narcolepsy and Disruption to Social Functioning" (Culbertson & Bruck, 2005), from the School of Psychology at Victoria University in Melbourne, Australia, which gave patient quotes from 2005 that are very similar to what we are still struggling with almost twenty years later. Here are some of the interesting quotes from their publication:

"The hardest part is fitting in with the rest of the world. . ."

"Thirty-one years, and he still hasn't got it straight; he will walk in and give me a surprise and walk off, and I'm standing there grabbing hold of something, and he has walked off. He never even thinks to look." (describing cataplexy)

"I have a good friend . . . one person that really understands."

"It's very, very difficult. People invite me out for meals occasionally . . . it's just awful. They always get a nice warm room ready; they always get you a big meal, and it's just so conducive to going to sleep. It is so embarrassing . . . and that dreadful feeling of trying to stay awake. 'Oh, I mustn't go to sleep. I must try and stay awake, I must listen to what they're saying, I must talk to them and be sociable,' and all the time, I'm dropping off. It's just awful."

"(It's) frustrating that you don't see it. I know that people don't believe me. I would expect them not to believe; it's too bizarre."

"I know there are other illnesses that are so much more grave and life-threatening than mine, but in many of these, the public knowledge is so much better. Understanding and acceptance are there."

"I want to have a life; I want to have respect and do something for myself. I'm sick, okay, I understand that, but this is not a disease I can't manage. I could have a very well-oriented career with this disease and be able to be successful . . ."

Hypersomnia/Excessive Daytime Sleepiness Quotes I Have Collected from My Patients Throughout the Years

"I can go to sleep with a snap of a finger."

"I could nap anywhere, anytime. I take my lunch, and I nap. Immediately after work, I nap . . . I have to."

"I used to fall asleep while sitting in traffic or while speaking after returning home from work."

"It really affects my recall and memory in the afternoon."

"Sometimes I feel drunk for a while after I wake up."

"I have difficulty getting ready in the morning; I can't wake up."

"Daytime sleepiness causes irritability—it's difficult to do any task without being irritable."

"People always poke fun at me for napping—implying I'm lazy."

"No one in my extended family understands my Narcolepsy, and they say hurtful things."

"People tell me I just need to have a cup of coffee and not a nap . . ."

"I have a lot of guilt because of my sleepiness and the Narcolepsy limits."

"Everyone notices she sleeps a lot."

"I yawn all the time in the evening . . . once I start, I can't stop."

"I put my car in park at all red lights, drive-thru windows, and anytime I am stopped. I figure a horn blow behind me is better than a crash in front of me—I've had fender benders."

"I don't drive very long at all because I am so sleepy."

"I never wake up rested."

"I am constantly moving because if I sit down, I fall asleep."

"I can sleep while trying to maintain a conversation."

"When I am sleepy, my brain feels full."

"There are these gaps." (Micro sleeps)

"When I get stressed, it is like giving me something to make me sleep."

"When things get bad, I just have to go to bed."

"I have had a few minor wrecks because I am so sleepy."

"My family always commented I was lazy or faking it, being so tired."

"I had to pull over and nap on the way to school after having slept all night."

"My friends have pointed out I always say I'm tired."

"I have had three accidents in one month from falling asleep at the wheel. I had to stop driving."

"I have fallen asleep driving, even with Adderall."

"This affects our lives negatively. She has trouble getting to almost anything on time, as she has to make time for sleep."

"I turn my alarm off in my sleep. I must have someone call me every morning to wake me up."

"This impairs my ability to have an orgasm . . . I'm so sleepy."

"With emotions, I get very tired."

"I have fallen asleep while standing up and brushing my teeth."

"I fall asleep at my computer at work."

"I don't get time for naps anymore, so I go to bed at about 7:00 p.m."

"Sometimes it is really hard for me to wake up from my naps."

"I fall asleep at school, at home after school, and I can't do my homework. I am so sleepy."

"I don't like to eat because every time I eat, I have to lie down to take a nap."

"I will fall asleep at red lights and while standing up in my clinical rotations."

"I'm too tired to take care of myself."

"I'm lifeless—it's like I'm in another world."

"I have jumbled words, and my comprehension is not good when sleepy."

"I have fallen asleep while standing up."

"It takes three alarms to get up, and sometimes I oversleep." (This patient even tried going to the meeting place for work and sleeping in his truck to avoid being late.)

"I set ten alarm clocks to get up. It's like I'm in this quicksand pit—I'm exhausted, and I don't know if I can get myself out."

"My friends take pictures of me falling asleep in class and when we are out."

"My hands don't work well."

"I've had wrecks, cuts on my head from falling during cataplexy, job loss, and loss of a relationship due to Narcolepsy. I feel worthless."

"The only thing that helps me when I'm sleepy is to take a nap."

"I've never been a high-energy person, but at eighteen, I started napping . . . I had to."

"I feel like I'm running in place. I'm slow at everything. I'm exhausted all the time."

"Being tired during the day without any relief."

"Sleeping during conversations . . . my husband gets mad."

"Sex. . . sex is impaired because I am so sleepy all the time."

"The exhaustion leaves me overwhelmed, moody, and easily frustrated."

"She has fallen asleep at concerts while the bands are playing."

"She often misses activities during the day due to napping excessively—every day."

"I've noticed increased sleepiness in high-stress situations (finals)."

"I think about napping all the time."

"My brain is foggy."

"I lost my long-term job because I can't get up in the morning and am always late."

"I have relationship issues due to always being out of it."

"I have issues completing the simplest of daily tasks that need to be done."

"Driving forty-five minutes to my office can be scary!"

"When driving, I MUST have meds."

"I have difficulty when the schedule needs to be changed—routine helps."

"I have a lot of alarms that I sometimes shut off unknowingly."

"It's not every day, but some days are worse than others."

"Although I need naps, sometimes it is hard to wake up from them, so I won't take them."

"My husband resents me and my health problems."

"I'm too sleepy sometimes, but not all the time for sex."

"It gets really hard if I am waiting on hold on the phone, helping my kids with homework, in long meetings . . ."

"People always poke fun at me for my napping, implying that I'm lazy. That is hurtful."

"I get so sleepy it is painful."

"I crave sleep. It gets better with treatment, but I crave sleep."

"This has caused problems in multiple relationships."

"I have trouble paying attention because I'm so sleepy and thinking about naps."

"My family does not like me being too sleepy to do things with them."

"My life has no discipline because my sleep habits are so erratic. I am a slave to them."

Cataplexy = Muscle Weakness with Emotions

"Something that I did not notice was cataplexy. I had it. I did not know what it was or even that it was abnormal. Now, I know."

A patient with a fear of heights once reported that his knees buckled when he got on a high diving board at the swimming pool. This was one of the first times he realized he had cataplexy.

"I start stuttering with extreme sleepiness."

"My legs give out."

"I melt when I laugh, mostly in my thighs."

"Sometimes I stutter, mostly when I am excited."

"I have balance problems due to sleepiness."

"I have droopy eyelids sometimes and cannot raise them."

"I sometimes have a shaking sensation in my brain when I feel emotional."

"I am insanely clumsy."

"I have such anxiety about spilling my Xyrem that I have cataplexy and spill my Xyrem."

"My whole body gets weak with laughter."

"Extremes in heat can cause me to lose strength in my arms too, and I can't lift as much."

"I don't laugh anymore; I don't even talk much. I'm like a shell of myself. I try to avoid the cataplexy."

"I have cataplexy with negative emotions; when I'm anxious, overwhelmed, or exacerbated . . . my arms and chest feel heavy

like I can't hold my body up . . . I feel weak . . .
I have to take a nap."

"Sometimes her legs get too weak to walk."

"I have more symptoms now, but Wakix helps—just lots of
emotions and bad news right now."

"I drop my pencil."

"I once fell while fighting with my girlfriend walking up the
stairs. I hit my head and had to have stitches."

"I drop my cell phone every time I laugh.
I have had multiple cell phones!"

"I fall on the grass when walking
across campus and my friends tell a joke."

"Her face looks funny when she hears something funny;
it's off balance."

"It's almost like Bell's Palsy in my face when
I get really upset."

"The cataplexy's usually in my right knee and legs.
I can hardly stand."

Sleep Paralysis Quotes

"I'm lost in my body . . . like I can't move."

"It's like my arms are weak, but my legs weigh a ton, and I just
have to wait until everything evens out before I can get up."

"Like a dark force holding me down."

"I have sleep paralysis most nights and with most naps when I
fall asleep."

"It is like sleep drowning. Have you ever been on the lake and are right under the water and feel like you cannot pull yourself out for a minute?"

Hypnogogic Hallucinations

"I'm not crazy, am I? I hear doors shut when I am going to sleep."

"I will not nap due to the hypnagogic hallucinations, which lead to panic."

"It's like it is happening in real life as I'm going to sleep."

"I can dream before my brain shuts down."

"It is like I can feel someone or something touching me lightly."

"I see a shadow as I am going to sleep."

"Sometimes I hear music when I go to sleep or wake up."

Disrupted Nocturnal Sleep

"I feel like my dreams are super, super real when I wake up."

"I'm sleepy, and then when I lay down at night, I can't sleep."

"I'm sleeping, but I don't feel rested."

"I have severe nightmares!"

"I feel like I have to work to get to sleep and get so frustrated at night!"

"Not sleeping is horrible when you are so sleepy."

"I get so worried about not sleeping that I can't sleep."

"Since I'm sleeping better, the Narcolepsy isn't as bad."

"I'm just barely under when I sleep."

"Sleep, or the lack thereof, dictates my daily activities and whether I can function."

Interesting Things on the Internet About Narcolepsy

"If one has both insomnia and Narcolepsy, do they cancel each other out?" Quickmeme.com

"Oh, you have Narcolepsy. Please tell me about the awesome places you've slept." Frabz.com

"You won't feel sleepy at work . . . if you sleep at work." healthline.com

"Cataplexy: When emotions paralyze you." i.9.qizmodo.com

"My day starts backward. I wake up tired and go to bed wide awake." Pinterest

"Feeling like my limbs are overcooked spaghetti." r/Narcolepsy post on Reddit

"Morning: Tired. Afternoon: Dying for a nap. Night: Can't Sleep." A Pea in the Pod

"I'm sorry for what I said when you tried to wake me up." thenapmistress on Instagram

"My dreams are extremely realistic. Sometimes I can't tell the difference. I feel everything in the waking world . . . all the senses and stuff. Even pain at times." Project Sleep, 2023, "Narcolepsy and Art" Podcast by Jayden Rowland

"Narcolepsy: When a nap is about as refreshing as eight hours of sleep, and eight hours of sleep is as refreshing as a nap." Pinterest

Afterword

Waking to a New Day!

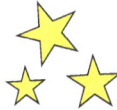

IT'S NOT A DREAM, IT'S A PLAN

*"Good night—may you fall asleep in the
arms of a dream so beautiful you'll cry when you awake."*
Micahel Faudet

Hopefully, this book has inspired you, answered some of your questions, and told you where to look for others. In the words of Lao Tzu, "The journey of a thousand miles begins with one step." Take the first step. Get started!

Make notes. Use the action plan attached to this book. Consider making it a yearly New Year's resolution to reread this book or something like it each January to start your New Year's journey and make any adjustments you may need to your plan.

Monitor your progress and look for areas where you may need help to improve your symptoms, as they may change over time. Retake the NAPS questionnaire periodically (maybe several times a year). Share the results with your provider. Monitor for new research and new treatments available to you. Be aggressive in finding all available options and opportunities out there. You are the captain of your team; don't wait for providers to update you.

Share your knowledge! As I said before, knowledge is power! You can now help someone else in their journey to identify their Narcolepsy and what they can do to get help. Please get involved in support groups, the Narcolepsy Network, Project Sleep, Wake Up Narcolepsy, or any other organizations I have mentioned. They really can be helpful. Help your family understand you and this disorder.

In her book, on page 180, Julie Flygare said, "But I had a secret weapon—an illness that had taken me to the ground and stripped me of my athleticism. I now realized this was not time wasted but time spent building me into the person and runner I would become. Narcolepsy had become a source of inspiration—helping me to live in the moment with immediacy and gratitude. Strange as it may sound, sickness was my second chance."

May your Narcolepsy journey help you discover a second chance full of gratitude, living in the moment, and unlimited possibilities! Light the fire and spread the word!

Best of Luck to You!

Debra J. Stultz, M.D.

*"Always remember that your present situation
is not your final destination.*

The best is yet to come!"

Zig Ziglar

References

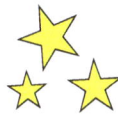

Abad, V., & Guilleminault, C. (2017). New developments in the management of narcolepsy. *Nature and Science of Sleep, Volume 9*, 39–57. https://doi.org/10.2147/NSS.S103467

Acquavella, J., Mehra, R., Bron, M., Suomi, J. M.-H., & Hess, G. P. (2020). Prevalence of narcolepsy and other sleep disorders and frequency of diagnostic tests from 2013–2016 in insured patients actively seeking care. *Journal of Clinical Sleep Medicine, 16*(8), 1255–1263. https://doi.org/10.5664/jcsm.8482

Ajayi, S., Kinagi, R., & Haslett, E. (2012). Obstetric Management of a Patient with Narcolepsy and Cataplexy: A Case Report. *Case Reports in Obstetrics and Gynecology, 2012*, 1–2. https://doi.org/10.1155/2012/982039

American Academy of Sleep Medicine. International Classification of Sleep Disorders, 3rd ed. (2014). American Academy of Sleep Disorder.

American Psychiatric Association. (2013). *Diagnostic and Statistical Manual of Mental Disorders*. American Psychiatric Association. https://doi.org/10.1176/appi.books.9780890425596

Anic-Labat, S., Guilleminault, C., Kraemer, H. C., Meehan, J., Arrigoni, J., & Mignot, E. (1999a). Validation of a cataplexy questionnaire in 983 sleep-disorders patients. *Sleep, 22*(1), 77–87. https://doi.org/10.1139/X08-079

Anic-Labat, S., Guilleminault, C., Kraemer, H. C., Meehan, J., Arrigoni, J., & Mignot, E. (1999b). Validation of a cataplexy questionnaire in 983 sleep-disorders patients. *Sleep, 22*(1), 77–87. http://www.ncbi.nlm.nih.gov/pubmed/9989368

BaHammam, A., Alnakshabandi, K., & Pandi-Perumal, S., (2020). Neuropsychiatric Correlates of Narcolepsy. *Current Psychiatry Reports.* Springer. https://doi.org/10.1007/s11920-020-01159-y

Bayard, S., Lanenier, M.D., De Cock, V.C., Scholz, S., & Dauvilliers, Y. (2012). Executive control of attention in narcolepsy. *PLoS ONE, 7*(4), e33525. https://doi.org/https://psycnet.apa.org/doi/10.1371/journal.pone.0033525

Benmedjahed, K., Wang, Y. G., Lambert, J., Evans, C., Hwang, S., Black, J., & Johns, M. W. (2017). Assessing sleepiness and cataplexy in children and adolescents with narcolepsy: a review of current patient-reported measures. *Sleep Medicine, 32,* 143–149. https://doi.org/10.1016/j.sleep.2016.12.020

Black, J., Reaven, N. L., Funk, S. E., McGaughey, K., Ohayon, M. M., Guilleminault, C., & Ruoff, C. (2017). Medical comorbidity in narcolepsy: findings from the Burden of Narcolepsy Disease (BOND) study. *Sleep Medicine, 33,* 13–18. https://doi.org/10.1016/j.sleep.2016.04.004

Bogan, R., Stern, T., Corser, B., Franco, J., Konofal, E., Apostol, G., Morse, A., Kushida, C., Thorpy, M., & Rosenberg, R. (2023). 0578 Clinician and Patient Global Impression in a Phase 2 Study of Mazindol (NLS-1021) in Adults with Narcolepsy Type 1 and Type 2. *SLEEP, 46*(Supplement_1), A254–A254. https://doi.org/10.1093/sleep/zsad077.0578

Bray, N. (2018). A narcotic–narcoleptic link. *Nature Reviews Neuroscience, 19*(9), 518–518. https://doi.org/10.1038/s41583-018-0043-y

Calvo-Ferrandiz, E., & Peraita-Adrados, R. (2018). Narcolepsy with cataplexy and pregnancy: a case-control study. *Journal of Sleep Research,* 27(2), 270–274. https://doi.org/10.1111/jsr.12567

Carskadon, M. A. (1986a). Guidelines for the Multiple Sleep Latency Test (MSLT): A Standard Measure of Sleepiness. *Sleep, 9*(4), 519–524. https://doi.org/10.1093/sleep/9.4.519

Carskadon, M. A. (1986b). Guidelines for the Multiple Sleep Latency Test (MSLT): A Standard Measure of Sleepiness. *Sleep, 9*(4), 519–524. https://doi.org/10.1093/sleep/9.4.519

Case Book of Sleep Medicine, Third Edition (Third Edit). (2019). American Academy of Sleep Medicine.

Chakravorty, S. S., & Rye, D. B. (2003). Narcolepsy in the Older Adult. *Drugs & Aging*, 20(5), 361–376. https://doi.org/10.2165/00002512-200320050-00005

Cheung, J., Ruoff, C. M., & Mignot, E. (2017). Central Nervous System Hypersomnias. In *Sleep and Neurologic Disease* (pp. 141–166). Elsevier. https://doi.org/10.1016/B978-0-12-804074-4.00008-X

Culbertson, H., & Bruck, D. (2005). Narcolepsy and Disruption to Social Functioning. *E-Journal of Applied Psychology*, 1(1), 14–22. https://doi.org/10.7790/ejap.v1i1.5

Dauvilliers, Y., Chen, A., Whalen, M., Macfadden, W., & Thorpy, M. (2023). 0592 Efficacy of Lower-Sodium Oxybate by Baseline Sleep Inertia in a Phase 3 Clinical Study in Patients With Idiopathic Hypersomnia. *SLEEP*, 46(Supplement_1), A260–A260. https://doi.org/10.1093/sleep/zsad077.0592

Dauvilliers, Y., Montplaisir, J., Molinari, N., Carlander, B., Ondze, B., Besset, A., & Billiard, M. (2001). Age at onset of narcolepsy in two large populations of patients in France and Quebec. *Neurology*, 57(11), 2029–2033. https://doi.org/10.1212/WNL.57.11.2029

Davidson, R. D., Biddle, K., Nassan, M., Scammell, T. E., & Zhou, E. S. (2022). The impact of narcolepsy on social relationships in young adults. *Journal of Clinical Sleep Medicine*, 18(12), 2751–2761. https://doi.org/10.5664/jcsm.10212

Davis, J. L., & Wright, D. C. (2006). Exposure, Relaxation, and Rescripting Treatment for Trauma-Related Nightmares. *Journal of Trauma & Dissociation*, 7(1), 5–18. https://doi.org/10.1300/J229v07n01_02

de Martin Truzzi, G., Naufel, M. F., Tufik, S., & Coelho, F. M. (2020). The influence of narcolepsy on olfactory function: a review. *Sleep Medicine*, 72, 75–81. https://doi.org/10.1016/j.sleep.2020.03.023

Deak, M., & Epstein, L. J. (2009). The History of Polysomnography. *Sleep Medicine Clinics*, 4(3), 313–321. https://doi.org/10.1016/j.jsmc.2009.04.001

Drake, C., Nickel, C., Burduvali, E., Roth, T., Jefferson, C., & Pietro, B. (2003). The pediatric daytime sleepiness scale (PDSS): sleep habits and school outcomes in middle-school children. *Sleep*, *26*(4), 455–458. http://www.ncbi.nlm.nih.gov/pubmed/12841372

Elliott, L., & Swick, T. (2015). Treatment paradigms for cataplexy in narcolepsy: past, present, and future. *Nature and Science of Sleep*, 159. https://doi.org/10.2147/NSS.S92140

Flygare, J. (2012). *Wide Awake and Dreaming: A Memoir*. Mill Pond Swan Publishing.

Franceschini, C., Pizza, F., Cavalli, F., & Plazzi, G. (2021). A practical guide to the pharmacological and behavioral therapy of Narcolepsy. *Neurotherapeutics*, *18*(1), 6–19. https://doi.org/10.1007/s13311-021-01051-4

Frauscher, B., Ehrmann, L., Mitterling, T., Gabelia, D., Gschliesser, V., Brandauer, E., Poewe, W., & Högl, B. (2013). Delayed Diagnosis, Range of Severity, and Multiple Sleep Comorbidities: A Clinical and Polysomnographic Analysis of 100 Patients of the Innsbruck Narcolepsy Cohort. *Journal of Clinical Sleep Medicine*, *09*(08), 805–812. https://doi.org/10.5664/jcsm.2926

Hamid, M., Franco, R., & Battistini, H. (2020). STATUS CATAPLECTICUS INDUCED BY WITHDRAWAL OF DULOXETINE. *Chest*, *158*(4), A2315. https://doi.org/10.1016/j.chest.2020.08.1965

Heidbreder, A., Dirks, C., & Ramm, M. (2020). Therapy for Cataplexy. *Current Treatment Options in Neurology*, *22*(4), 13. https://doi.org/10.1007/s11940-020-0619-5

Hoddes, E., Zarcone, V., Smythe, H., Phillips, R., & Dement, W. C. (1973). Quantification of Sleepiness: A New Approach. *Psychophysiology*, *10*(4), 431–436. https://doi.org/10.1111/j.1469-8986.1973.tb00801.x

HUBLIN, C., KAPRIO, J., PARTINEN, M., KOSKENVUO, M., & HEIKKILÄ, K. (1994). The Ullanlinna Narcolepsy Scale: validation of a measure of symptoms in the narcoleptic syndrome. *Journal of Sleep Research*, *3*(1), 52–59. https://doi.org/10.1111/j.1365-2869.1994.tb00104.x

Hublin, C., Partinen, M., Heinonen, E. H., Puukka, P., & Salmi, T. (1994). Selegiline in the treatment of narcolepsy. *Neurology*, *44*(11), 2095–2095. https://doi.org/10.1212/WNL.44.11.2095

International Classification of Sleep Disorders (Third Edit). (2014). American Academy of Sleep Medicine.

Johns, M. W. (1991). A New Method for Measuring Daytime Sleepiness: The Epworth Sleepiness Scale. *Sleep*, *14*(6), 540–545. https://doi.org/10.1093/sleep/14.6.540

Jung, Y., & St. Louis, E. K. (2016). Treatment of REM Sleep Behavior Disorder. *Current Treatment Options in Neurology*, *18*(11), 50. https://doi.org/10.1007/s11940-016-0433-2

Kim, J., Lee, G.-H., Sung, S. M., Jung, D. S., & Pak, K. (2020). Prevalence of attention deficit hyperactivity disorder symptoms in narcolepsy: a systematic review. *Sleep Medicine*, *65*, 84–88. https://doi.org/10.1016/j.sleep.2019.07.022

Krahn, L.E., Lymp, J.F., Moore, W.R., Slocumb N., S. M. H. (2005). Characterizing the emotions that trigger cataplexy. *J. Neuropsychiatry ClinNeuroscie,* 17(1), 45–50. https://doi.org/10.1176/ jnp.17.1.45

Krahn, L.E.; Arand, D.L.; Avidan, A.Y.; Davilla, D. G.; DeBassio, W. A.; Ruoff, C. M.; Harrod, C. G. (2021). Recommended protocols for the Multiple Sleep Latency Test and Maintenance of Wakefulness Test in adults: quidance from the American Academy of Sleep Medicine. *Journal of Clinical Sleep Medicine*, *17*(12). https://doi.org/10.5664/jcsm.9620

Krakow, B., Kellner, R., Pathak, D., & Lambert, L. (1995). Imagery rehearsal treatment for chronic nightmares. *Behaviour Research and Therapy*, *33*(7), 837–843. https://doi.org/10.1016/0005-7967(95)00009-M

Lankford, D. A., Wellman, J. J., & O'Hara, C. (1994). Posttraumatic Narcolepsy in Mild to Moderate Closed Head Injury. *Sleep*, *17*(suppl_8), S25–S28. https://doi.org/10.1093/sleep/17.suppl_8.S25

Lu, M., Zhang, Y., Zhang, J., Huang, S., Huang, F., Wang, T., Wu, F., Mao, H., & Huang, Z. (2023). Comparative Effectiveness of Digital Cognitive Behavioral Therapy vs Medication Therapy Among Patients With Insomnia. *JAMA Network Open*, *6*(4), e237597. https://doi.org/10.1001/jamanetworkopen.2023.7597

Marín Agudelo, H. A., Jiménez Correa, U., Carlos Sierra, J., Pandi-Perumal, S. R., & Schenck, C. H. (2014). Cognitive behavioral treatment for narcolepsy: can it complement pharmacotherapy? *Sleep Science*, *7*(1), 30–42. https://doi.org/10.1016/j.slsci.2014.07.023

Martínez-Rodríguez, J. E., Iranzo, A., Santamaría, J., Genís, D., Molins, A., Silva, Y., & Meléndez, R. (2002). [Status cataplecticus induced by abrupt withdrawal of clomipramine]. *Neurologia (Barcelona, Spain)*, *17*(2), 113–116. http://www.ncbi.nlm.nih.gov/pubmed/11864561

Maski, K., Mignot, E., Plazzi, G., & Dauvilliers, Y. (2022). Disrupted nighttime sleep and sleep instability in narcolepsy. *Journal of Clinical Sleep Medicine*, *18*(1), 289–304. https://doi.org/10.5664/jcsm.9638

Maski, K., Steinhart, E., Williams, D., Scammell, T., Flygare, J., McCleary, K., & Gow, M. (2017). Listening to the Patient Voice in Narcolepsy: Diagnostic Delay, Disease Burden, and Treatment Efficacy. *Journal of Clinical Sleep Medicine*, *13*(03), 419–425. https://doi.org/10.5664/jcsm.6494

Mitchell, M. D., Gehrman, P., Perlis, M., & Umscheid, C. A. (2012). Comparative effectiveness of cognitive behavioral therapy for insomnia: a systematic review. *BMC Family Practice*, *13*(1), 40. https://doi.org/10.1186/1471-2296-13-40

Mitler, M. M., Gujavarty, K. S., & Browman, C. P. (1982). Maintenance of wakefulness test: a polysomnographic technique for evaluation treatment efficacy in patients with excessive somnolence. *Electroencephalography and Clinical Neurophysiology*, *53*(6), 658–661. https://doi.org/10.1016/0013-4694(82)90142-0

Moore, W. R., Silber, M. H., Decker, P. A., Heim-Penokie, P. C., Sikkink, V. K., Slocumb[1], N., Richardson, J. W., & Krahn, L. E. (2007). Cataplexy Emotional Trigger Questionnaire (CETQ) — A Brief Patient Screen to Identify Cataplexy in Patients With Narcolepsy. *Journal of Clinical Sleep Medicine*, *03*(01), 37–40. https://doi.org/10.5664/jcsm.26743

Morgenthaler, T. I., Auerbach, S., Casey, K. R., Kristo, D., Maganti, R., Ramar, K., Zak, R., & Kartje, R. (2018). Position Paper for the Treatment of Nightmare Disorder in Adults: An American Academy of Sleep Medicine Position Paper. *Journal of Clinical Sleep Medicine*, *14*(06), 1041–1055. https://doi.org/10.5664/jcsm.7178

Morin, C. M. (2020). Cognitive behavioural therapy for insomnia (CBTi): From randomized controlled trials to practice guidelines to implementation in clinical practice. *Journal of Sleep Research*, *29*(2). https://doi.org/10.1111/jsr.13017

Morin, C. M., Vallières, A., Guay, B., Ivers, H., Savard, J., Mérette, C., Bastien, C., & Baillargeon, L. (2009). Cognitive Behavioral Therapy,

Singly and Combined With Medication, for Persistent Insomnia. *JAMA*, *301*(19), 2005. https://doi.org/10.1001/jama.2009.682

Morse, A. M. (2019). Narcolepsy in Children and Adults: A Guide to Improved Recognition, Diagnosis and Management. *Medical Sciences*, *7*(12), 106. https://doi.org/10.3390/medsci7120106

Morse, A. M., Kelly-Pieper, K., & Kothare, S. V. (2019). Management of Excessive Daytime Sleepiness in Narcolepsy With Baclofen. *Pediatric Neurology*, *93*, 39–42. https://doi.org/10.1016/j.pediatrneurol.2018.10.020

Morse, A., & Sanjeev, K. (2018). Narcolepsy and Psychiatric Disorders: Comorbidities or Shared Pathophysiology? *Medical Sciences*, *6*(1), 16. https://doi.org/10.3390/medsci6010016

Nishino, S. (2017). Cataplexy ☆. In *Reference Module in Neuroscience and Biobehavioral Psychology*. Elsevier. https://doi.org/10.1016/B978-0-12-809324-5.02137-4

Naumann, A.; Bellebaum, C.; Daum, I. (2006). Cognitive deficits in narcolepsy. *Journal of Sleep Research*, *15*(3), 329–338. https://doi.org/https://doi.org/10.1111/j.1365-2869.2006.00533.x

Neikrug, A. B., Crawford, M. R., & Ong, J. C. (2017). Behavioral Sleep Medicine Services for Hypersomnia Disorders: A Survey Study. *Behavioral Sleep Medicine*, *15*(2), 158–171. https://doi.org/10.1080/15402002.2015.1120201

Nightingale, S., Orgill, J. C., Ebrahim, I. O., de Lacy, S. F., Agrawal, S., & Williams, A. J. (2005). The association between narcolepsy and REM behavior disorder (RBD). *Sleep Medicine*, *6*(3), 253–258. https://doi.org/10.1016/j.sleep.2004.11.007

Ohayon, M. M. (2013). Narcolepsy is complicated by high medical and psychiatric comorbidities: a comparison with the general population. *Sleep Medicine*, *14*(6), 488–492. https://doi.org/10.1016/j.sleep.2013.03.002

Ohayon, M. M., Thorpy, M. J., Carls, G., Black, J., Cisternas, M., Pasta, D. J., Bujanover, S., Hyman, D., & Villa, K. F. (2021). The Nexus Narcolepsy Registry: methodology, study population characteristics, and patterns and predictors of narcolepsy diagnosis. *Sleep Medicine*, *84*, 405–414. https://doi.org/10.1016/j.sleep.2021.06.008

Omari, N. B., & Kinyungu, N. M. (2022). Reduced Cataplexy Symptoms While on Suboxone: A Case Report. *Journal of Behavioral and Brain Science*, *12*(11), 548–551. https://doi.org/10.4236/jbbs.2022.1211032

Ong, J. C., Dawson, S. C., Mundt, J. M., & Moore, C. (2020). Developing a cognitive behavioral therapy for hypersomnia using telehealth: a feasibility study. *Journal of Clinical Sleep Medicine*, *16*(12), 2047–2062. https://doi.org/10.5664/jcsm.8750

Overeem, S., van Nues, S. J., van der Zande, W. L., Donjacour, C. E., van Mierlo, P., & Lammers, G. J. (2011a). The clinical features of cataplexy: A questionnaire study in narcolepsy patients with and without hypocretin-1 deficiency. *Sleep Medicine*, *12*(1), 12–18. https://doi.org/10.1016/j.sleep.2010.05.010

Overeem, S., van Nues, S. J., van der Zande, W. L., Donjacour, C. E., van Mierlo, P., & Lammers, G. J. (2011b). The clinical features of cataplexy: A questionnaire study in narcolepsy patients with and without hypocretin-1 deficiency. *Sleep Medicine*, *12*(1), 12–18. https://doi.org/10.1016/j.sleep.2010.05.010

Palhano, A.C.M; Kim, L.J.; Moreira, G. A.; Coelho, F. M.; Tufik, S. (2018). Narcolepsy, Precocious Puberty and Obesity in the Pediatric Population: a Literature Review. *Pediatric Endocruinology Reviews*, *16*(2), 266–274. https://doi.org/10.17458/per.vol16.2018. Narcolepsypubertyobesity

Pelayo R, L. M. (2005). *Sleep: A Comprehensive Handbook*. (T. Lee-Chiong, Ed.). Wiley. https://doi.org/10.1002/0471751723

Pellitteri, G., Dolso, P., Valente, M., & Gigli, G. L. (2020). Orgasmolepsy in Narcolepsy Type 1 Responsive to Pitolisant: A Case Report. *Nature and Science of Sleep*, *Volume 12*, 1237–1240. https://doi.org/10.2147/NSS.S286358

Pereira, D., Lopes, E., da Silva Behrens, N. S. C., de Almeida Fonseca, H., Sguillar, D. A., de Araújo Lima, T. F., Pradella-Hallinan, M., Castro, J., Tufik, S., & Santos Coelho, F. M. (2014). Prevalence of periodical leg movements in patients with narcolepsy in an outpatient facility in São Paulo. *Sleep Science*, *7*(1), 69–71. https://doi.org/10.1016/j.slsci.2014.07.018

Pillen, S., Pizza, F., Dhondt, K., Scammell, T. E., & Overeem, S. (2017). Cataplexy and Its Mimics: Clinical Recognition and Management. *Current Treatment Options in Neurology*, *19*(6), 23. https://doi.org/10.1007/s11940-017-0459-0

Ping, L. S., Yat, F. S. Y., & Kwok, W. Y. (2007). Status cataplecticus leading to the obstetric complication of prolonged labor. *Journal of Clinical Sleep Medicine : JCSM : Official Publication of the American Academy of Sleep Medicine, 3*(1), 56–57. http://www.ncbi.nlm.nih.gov/pubmed/17557454

Pizza, F., Antelmi, E., Vandi, S., Meletti, S., Erro, R., Baumann, C. R., Bhatia, K. P., Dauvilliers, Y., Edwards, M. J., Iranzo, A., Overeem, S., Tinazzi, M., Liguori, R., & Plazzi, G. (2018). The distinguishing motor features of cataplexy: a study from video-recorded attacks. *Sleep, 41*(5). https://doi.org/10.1093/sleep/zsy026

Plazzi, G., Clawges, H. M., & Owens, J. A. (2018). Clinical Characteristics and Burden of Illness in Pediatric Patients with Narcolepsy. *Pediatric Neurology, 85*, 21–32. https://doi.org/10.1016/j.pediatrneurol.2018.06.008

Quaedackers, L., Pillen, S., & Overeem, S. (2021). Recognizing the Symptom Spectrum of Narcolepsy to Improve Timely Diagnosis: A Narrative Review. *Nature and Science of Sleep, Volume 13*, 1083–1096. https://doi.org/10.2147/NSS.S278046

Rosenberg, R., Citrome, L., & Drake, C. L. (2021). Advances in the Treatment of Chronic Insomnia: A Narrative Review of New Nonpharmacologic and Pharmacologic Therapies. *Neuropsychiatric Disease and Treatment, Volume 17*, 2549–2566. https://doi.org/10.2147/NDT.S297504

Roth, T., Dauvilliers, Y., Mignot, E., Montplaisir, J., Paul, J., Swick, T., & Zee, P. (2013). Disrupted Nighttime Sleep in Narcolepsy. *Journal of Clinical Sleep Medicine, 09*(09), 955–965. https://doi.org/10.5664/jcsm.3004

Ruoff, C. M., Reaven, N. L., Funk, S. E., McGaughey, K. J., Ohayon, M. M., Guilleminault, C., & Black, J. (2017). High Rates of Psychiatric Comorbidity in Narcolepsy. *The Journal of Clinical Psychiatry, 78*(02), 171–176. https://doi.org/10.4088/JCP.15m10262

Sandsmark, D. K., Elliott, J. E., & Lim, M. M. (2017). Sleep-Wake Disturbances After Traumatic Brain Injury: Synthesis of Human and Animal Studies. *Sleep.* https://doi.org/10.1093/sleep/zsx044

Sansa, G., Iranzo, A., & Santamaria, J. (2010). Obstructive sleep apnea in narcolepsy. *Sleep Medicine, 11*(1), 93–95. https://doi.org/10.1016/j.sleep.2009.02.009

Scammell, T. E. (2015). Narcolepsy. *New England Journal of Medicine*, *373*(27), 2654–2662. https://doi.org/10.1056/NEJMra1500587

Scammell, T. E. (2023). Treatment of narcolepsy in adults. In *UpToDate*. www.uptodate.com

Scammell, T. E., Luo, G., Borker, P., Sullivan, L., Biddle, K., & Mignot, E. (2020). Treatment of narcolepsy with natalizumab. *Sleep*, *43*(7). https://doi.org/10.1093/sleep/zsaa050

Scheer, D., Schwartz, S. W., Parr, M., Zgibor, J., Sanchez-Anguiano, A., & Rajaram, L. (2019). Prevalence and incidence of narcolepsy in a US health care claims database, 2008–2010. *Sleep*, *42*(7). https://doi.org/10.1093/sleep/zsz091

Schneider, L.; and Ellenbogen, J. (2020). Images: Facial cataplexy with demonstration of persistent eye movement. *J Clin Sleep Med*, 16(1),157–159. https://doi.org/https:/jcsm.8148

Serra, L., Montagna, P., Mignot, E., Lugaresi, E., & Plazzi, G. (2008a). Cataplexy features in childhood narcolepsy. *Movement Disorders*, *23*(6), 858–865. https://doi.org/10.1002/mds.21965

Serra, L., Montagna, P., Mignot, E., Lugaresi, E., & Plazzi, G. (2008b). Cataplexy features in childhood narcolepsy. *Movement Disorders*, *23*(6), 858–865. https://doi.org/10.1002/mds.21965

Shahid, A., Wilkinson, K., Marcu, S., & Shapiro, C. M. (2011). Karolinska Sleepiness Scale (KSS). In *STOP, THAT and One Hundred Other Sleep Scales* (pp. 209–210). Springer New York. https://doi.org/10.1007/978-1-4419-9893-4_47

Spriggs, W. H. (2014). *Essentials of Polysomnography: A Training Guide and Reference for Sleep Technicians*. Jones & Barlett Learning.

Stultz, D., Osburn, S., Burns, T., Gills, T., Welch, D., Shaffer, C., Walton, R., Cope, A., & Pawlowska-Wajswol, S. (2021). 508 Narcolepsy Associated With a History of Head Injury: A Retrospective Review. *Sleep*, *44*(Supplement_2), A200–A200. https://doi.org/10.1093/sleep/zsab072.507

Sturzenegger, C.; Baumann, C.R.; Kallweith, U.; Lammers, G.J.; Bassetti, C. L. (2014). Swiss Narcolepsy Scale: a valid tool for the identification of hypocretin-1 deficient patients with narcolepsy. *Journal of Sleep Research*, *23*, 297. https://hdl.handle.net/1887/107166

Szakács, A., Hallböök, T., Tideman, P., Darin, N., & Wentz, E. (2015). Psychiatric Comorbidity and Cognitive Profile in Children with Narcolepsy with or without Association to the H1N1 Influenza Vaccination. *Sleep, 38*(4), 615–621. https://doi.org/10.5665/sleep.4582

Teixeira, V. G., Faccenda, J. F., & Douglas, N. J. (2004). Functional status in patients with narcolepsy. *Sleep Medicine*, 5(5), 477–483. https://doi.org/10.1016/j.sleep.2004.07.001

Thannickal, T. C., John, J., Shan, L., Swaab, D. F., Wu, M.-F., Ramanathan, L., McGregor, R., Chew, K.-T., Cornford, M., Yamanaka, A., Inutsuka, A., Fronczek, R., Lammers, G. J., Worley, P. F., & Siegel, J. M. (2018). Opiates increase the number of hypocretin-producing cells in human and mouse brain and reverse cataplexy in a mouse model of narcolepsy. *Science Translational Medicine, 10*(447). https://doi.org/10.1126/scitranslmed.aao4953

Thorpy, M. J. (2016a). Diagnostic Criteria and Delay in Diagnosis of Narcolepsy. In *Narcolepsy* (pp. 45–49). Springer International Publishing. https://doi.org/10.1007/978-3-319-23739-8_5

Thorpy, M. J. (2016b). Pregnancy and Anesthesia in Narcolepsy. In *Narcolepsy* (pp. 351–356). Springer International Publishing. https://doi.org/10.1007/978-3-319-23739-8_25

Thorpy, M. J. (2020a). Recently Approved and Upcoming Treatments for Narcolepsy. *CNS Drugs, 34*(1), 9–27. https://doi.org/10.1007/s40263-019-00689-1

Thorpy, M. J. (2020b). Recently Approved and Upcoming Treatments for Narcolepsy. *CNS Drugs, 34*(1), 9–27. https://doi.org/10.1007/s40263-019-00689-1

Thorpy, M. J., Hopper, J., & Patroneva, A. (2019). 0592 Burden of Narcolepsy: A Survey of Patients and Physicians. *Sleep, 42*(Supplement_1), A236–A236. https://doi.org/10.1093/sleep/zsz067.590

Thorpy, M. J., Shapiro, C., Mayer, G., Corser, B. C., Emsellem, H., Plazzi, G., Chen, D., Carter, L. P., Wang, H., Lu, Y., Black, J., & Dauvilliers, Y. (2019). A randomized study of solriamfetol for excessive sleepiness in narcolepsy. *Annals of Neurology, 85*(3), 359–370. https://doi.org/10.1002/ana.25423

Thorpy, M., Zhao, C. G., & Dauvilliers, Y. (2013). Management of narcolepsy during pregnancy. *Sleep Medicine, 14*(4), 367–376. https://doi.org/10.1016/j.sleep.2012.11.021

Van Dongen, H., Leary, E., Drake, C., Bogan, R., Jaeger, J., Rosenberg, R., Streicher, C., Kwak, H., Bates, J., & Tabuteau, H. (2023). 0559 Solriamfetol Demonstrates Durable Cognitive Improvement in Adults with Obstructive Sleep Apnea and Excessive Daytime Sleepiness. *SLEEP, 46*(Supplement_1), A246–A246. https://doi.org/10.1093/sleep/zsad077.0559

Vaughn, B. V., & D'Cruz, O. F. (1996). Carbamazepine as a Treatment for Cataplexy. *Sleep, 19*(2), 101–103. https://doi.org/10.1093/sleep/19.2.101

Wang, G., Benmedjahed, K., Lambert, J., Evans, C. J., Hwang, S., Black, J., & Johns, M. (2017). Assessing narcolepsy with cataplexy in children and adolescents: development of a cataplexy diary and the ESS-CHAD. *Nature and Science of Sleep, Volume 9*, 201–211. https://doi.org/10.2147/NSS.S140143

Wang, J., & Greenberg, H. (2013). Status Cataplecticus Precipitated by Abrupt Withdrawal of Venlafaxine. *Journal of Clinical Sleep Medicine, 09*(07), 715–716. https://doi.org/10.5664/jcsm.2848

Weaver, T. E., Pepin, J.-L., Schwab, R., Shapiro, C., Hedner, J., Ahmed, M., Foldvary-Schaefer, N., Strollo, P. J., Mayer, G., Sarmiento, K., Baladi, M., Bron, M., Chandler, P., Lee, L., & Malhotra, A. (2021). Long-term effects of solriamfetol on quality of life and work productivity in participants with excessive daytime sleepiness associated with narcolepsy or obstructive sleep apnea. *Journal of Clinical Sleep Medicine, 17*(10), 1995–2007. https://doi.org/10.5664/jcsm.9384

Wilson, A., Dongarwar, D., Carter, K., Marroquin, M., & Salihu, H. M. (2022). The association between narcolepsy during pregnancy and maternal-fetal risk factors/outcomes. *Sleep Science, 15*(3). https://doi.org/10.5935/1984-0063.20220054

Won, C., Mahmoudi, M., Qin, L., Purvis, T., Mathur, A., & Mohsenin, V. (2014). The Impact of Gender on Timeliness of Narcolepsy Diagnosis. *Journal of Clinical Sleep Medicine, 10*(01), 89–95. https://doi.org/10.5664/jcsm.3370

Xie, Z., Chen, F., Li, W. A., Geng, X., Li, C., Meng, X., Feng, Y., Liu, W., & Yu, F. (2017). A review of sleep disorders and melatonin. *Neurological Research, 39*(6), 559–565. https://doi.org/10.1080/01616412.2017.1315864

Zhang, M., Inocente, C. O., Villanueva, C., Lecendreux, M., Dauvilliers, Y., Lin, J., Arnulf, I., Gustin, M., Thieux, M., & Franco, P. (2020). Narcolepsy with cataplexy: Does age at diagnosis change the clinical picture? *CNS Neuroscience & Therapeutics, 26*(10), 1092–1102. https://doi.org/10.1111/cns.13438

Zhang, S., Ding, C., Wu, H., Fang, F., Wang, X., & Ren, X. (2015). [Clinical effect of atomoxetine hydrochloride in 66 children with narcolepsy]. *Zhonghua Er Ke Za Zhi = Chinese Journal of Pediatrics, 53*(10), 760–764. http://www.ncbi.nlm.nih.gov/pubmed/26758112

Appendix 1

Narcolepsy Assessment & Progress Screener

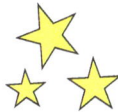

Adult Version

NAPS – P

Assessment & Progress Screener – Patient

Debra J. Stultz M.D., Laura B. Herpel M.D., and Lewis J. Kass M.D

Note: Completing this form thoughtfully and descriptively will help your evaluation and treatment plan.

1	In the last week, how would you rate your daytime sleepiness on a scale of 0 to 10 (with 10 being the most severe)?	
2	Typically, how would you rate your sleepiness throughout the day on a scale of 0 to 10 (with 10 being the most severe)?	
	a. Morning (8 AM – noon)	
	b. Afternoon (noon – 6 PM)	
	c. Evening (6 PM – 10 PM)	
3	To what extent do you avoid participating in social interactions because of your sleepiness or sleep disorder, on a scale of 0 to 10 (0 = no avoidance; 10 = most avoidance)?	
4	To what extent has your sleepiness or sleep disorder affected your abilities at work or school, on a scale of 0 to 10 (0 = not affected; 10 = most affected)?	
5	How many naps per day do you take?	

6	Cataplexy is any form of muscle weakness that occurs with strong emotion. Do you experience any of the following signs of cataplexy? (Check all that apply.)	
	<table><tr><td>• Facial weakness ☐</td><td>• Jaw weakness ☐</td></tr><tr><td>• Neck weakness ☐</td><td>• Arm weakness ☐</td></tr><tr><td>• Head dropping ☐</td><td>• Frequently dropping things ☐</td></tr><tr><td>• Blurred vision ☐</td><td></td></tr><tr><td>• Drooping eyelids ☐</td><td>• Frequent falls ☐</td></tr><tr><td>• Slurred speech ☐</td><td>• Being "clumsy" ☐</td></tr><tr><td>• Stuttering ☐</td><td>• Knees buckling ☐</td></tr><tr><td></td><td>• Ankles giving way ☐</td></tr></table>	
	The strong emotions causing this reaction can be laughter, anger, sadness, frustration, surprise, excitement, fear, sexual activity, humiliation, being caught off guard, or any other emotion.	
7	To what extent has cataplexy affected your ability to participate in social, work, and/or school activities on a scale of 0 to 10 (0 = not affected; 10 = most affected)?	
8	Do you have vivid dreams or nightmares? Yes ☐ No ☐ How often? _____	
9	Do you experience sleep paralysis, which is the sensation when waking up from sleep or falling asleep that your brain is awake, but you cannot move, or are your muscles (such as your hands) extremely weak when you first wake up? Yes ☐ No ☐ How often? _____	
10	Do you have any unusual experiences when falling asleep or waking up from sleep, such as seeing or hearing something that isn't really there or sensations as if you are immediately dreaming while going to sleep? Yes ☐ No ☐ How often? _____	

11	Do you have disrupted nighttime sleep with frequent awakenings or early morning awakenings? Yes ☐ No ☐ How often? _____
12	What strategies or medications have you found helpful for any of the above symptoms? _____ _____ _____
13	If you have started treatment for narcolepsy already, how would you rate your improvement on a scale of 0 to 10 (with 10 being the most improved)?
14	Please check any other sleep/mood/medicine-related issues you may be experiencing. a. Irregular sleep schedule ☐ b. Shift work ☐ c. Depression ☐ d. Anxiety ☐ e. Medications that cause sedation ☐ f. Sleeping more than 10 hours per night, with continued sleepiness during the day and long nap times ☐ g. History or symptoms of a head injury ☐ h. History or symptoms of sleep apnea (such as snoring and daytime sleepiness) ☐ Do you wear CPAP? Yes ☐ No ☐ If yes, how many nights per week? ___ i. Are there any other medical, psychiatric, or neurologic disorders that you feel may contribute to sleepiness? Yes ☐ No ☐ If yes, please describe. _____ _____ _____ _____

15	Have your family or friends commented on your degree of sleepiness, possible cataplexy, napping, or other related symptoms? Yes ☐ No ☐ If yes, please describe their concerns. _____ _____ _____ _____
16	Do you have any of the following issues? (Check all that apply.) a. Restless leg symptoms ☐ b. Kicking during sleep ☐ c. Sleepwalking/sleep talking/acting out dreams ☐ d. Having to get up at night to go to the bathroom ☐ e. Pets or children in the bed during sleep ☐ f. Bed partner with snoring or other issues that may disrupt your sleep ☐ g. Frequent accidents ☐
17	Please list 3 goals you hope to achieve with treatment.
	a.
	b.
	c.

NAPS – F

Narcolepsy Assessment & Progress Screener – Friends/Family

Patient name: _____

Your name: _____

Relationship to patient: _____

1. Have you noticed that your family member or friend experiences periods of excessive sleepiness during the daytime? Yes ☐ No ☐

2. Does it seem to you as if they nap more frequently than others? Yes ☐ No ☐

3. Have you ever noticed any unusual muscle weakness when they experience strong emotions? Examples of muscle weakness are facial drooping, slurred speech, neck weakness, falls, stuttering, drooping eyelids, dropping things, seeming clumsy, or knees buckling. Yes ☐ No ☐

4. Are you aware of any other family members who have been diagnosed with narcolepsy or are considered "sleepyheads"? Yes ☐ No ☐

5. Are there any areas of your family member or friend's life that you feel may be affected by extreme daytime sleepiness? Yes ☐ No ☐

6. If yes, please explain. _____

_____

_____

NAPS – C

Narcolepsy Assessment & Progress Screener – Clinician

Clinician/Patient Global Impression of Change (CGI-C)	

For each goal, please rate change since the previous visit using the following scale:
    +3 = significantly improved
    +2 = moderately improved
    +1 = mildly improved
    0 = no change
    -1 = mildly worse
    -2 = moderately worse
    -3 = significantly worse	

Goal	**Rating**

Current medications and doses:

Appendix 2

Narcolepsy Assessment & Progress Screener

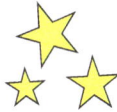

Pediatric Version

PED: NAPS

Pediatric Narcolepsy Assessment & Progress Screener

Debra J. Stultz M.D., Laura B. Herpel M.D., and Lewis J. Kass M.D

Patient name: _____ Date: _____

Your name: _____

Relationship to patient: _____

1	Has your child appeared sleepier recently? Yes ☐ No ☐
2	Does your child frequently complain of feeling sleepy? Yes ☐ No ☐
3	Is your child irritable at times, especially if sleepy? Yes ☐ No ☐
4	Does your child appear hyper at times, especially if sleepy? Yes ☐ No ☐
5	Is your child sleeping more than usual? Yes ☐ No ☐
6	Has your child fallen asleep in unusual places? Yes ☐ No ☐
7	Was your child "too good" of a sleeper in infancy? Yes ☐ No ☐
8	Was/is your child "too good" of a napper? Yes ☐ No ☐
9	Did your child start re-taking naps? Yes ☐ No ☐
10	Is your child a restless sleeper? Yes ☐ No ☐
11	Does your child snore? Yes ☐ No ☐

12	Is your child having issues at school with: _____ behavior _____ grades
13	Does your child fall asleep in school? Yes ☐ No ☐
14	Does your child have nap attacks, where they suddenly fall asleep? Yes ☐ No ☐
15	Does your child complain of nightmares or vivid dreams? Yes ☐ No ☐
16	Does your child have a history of a head injury? Yes ☐ No ☐
17	Does your child have trouble with concentration or memory? Yes ☐ No ☐
18	Has your child been diagnosed with ADHD? Yes ☐ No ☐
19	Is your child taking any medications for mood, anxiety, or ADHD? Yes ☐ No ☐
20	Has your child experienced a sudden onset of weight gain? Yes ☐ No ☐
21	Has your child missed school or social activities due to sleepiness? Yes ☐ No ☐
22	Does your child have any pets sleeping with them in bed? Yes ☐ No ☐
23	Does your child have a history of sleepwalking? Yes ☐ No ☐
24	Does your child ever complain of seeing or hearing things when falling asleep or waking up? Yes ☐ No ☐
25	Does your child ever complain that they cannot move briefly just after waking up? Yes ☐ No ☐

26	Muscle weakness – sudden loss of muscle control that is usually brief and temporary. Have you noticed your child having any of the following? (Check all that apply.)
	<table><tr><td>• Facial weakness ☐</td><td>• Knees buckling ☐</td></tr><tr><td>• Eyelid drooping ☐</td><td>• Decreased muscle</td></tr><tr><td>• Raised eyebrows ☐</td><td> tone ☐</td></tr><tr><td>• Jaw weakness ☐</td><td>• Being clumsy ☐</td></tr><tr><td>• Protruding tongue ☐</td><td>• Frequently dropping</td></tr><tr><td>• Tongue thrusting ☐</td><td> things ☐</td></tr><tr><td>• Grimacing ☐</td><td>• Frequent falls ☐</td></tr><tr><td>• Neck weakness ☐</td><td>• Frequent accidents ☐</td></tr><tr><td>• Neck extension ☐</td><td>• "Puppet-like"</td></tr><tr><td>• Head dropping or</td><td> movements ☐</td></tr><tr><td> bobbing ☐</td><td>• Slurred speech ☐</td></tr><tr><td>• Arm weakness ☐</td><td>• Stuttering ☐</td></tr></table>
27	Does your child fall down or get sleepy after getting the giggles? Yes ☐ No ☐
28	Does your child fall down or get sleepy after a tantrum? Yes ☐ No ☐
29	Does your child fall down or get sleepy after being surprised or shocked? Yes ☐ No ☐

30	Does your child have any of the following issues? (Check all that apply.)
	   a. Insomnia ☐
	   b. Restless legs before going to sleep ☐
	   c. Kicking during sleep ☐
	   d. Bedwetting ☐
	   e. Anxiety ☐
	   f. Depression ☐

31	Please list 3 ways you feel your child's sleep has impaired their ability to function.
	a.
	b.
	c.
32	Please list 3 goals you hope to achieve with treatment.
	a.
	b.
	c.

Appendix 3

Sleep and Psychiatric Medications

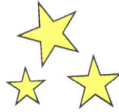

Brand Names and Generic Names for Medications Used in Narcolepsy

Misc Sleep

___ Mirapex (pramipexole)

___ Neupro Patch (rotigotine)

___ Nuvigil (armodafinil)

___ Provigil (modafinil)

___ Requip (ropinirole)

___ Wakix (pitolisant)

___ Xyrem (sodium oxybate)

___ Lumryz (sodium oxybate)

___ Xywav (calcium, magnesium, potassium, sodium oxybate)

___ Sunosi (solriamfetol)

Sleepers

___ Hetlioz (tasimelteon)

___ Quviviq (daridorexant)

Stimulants /Wake Promoting

___ Azstarys (serdexmethylphenidate)

___ Adzenys (amphetamine)

___ Adderall (amphetamine/ dextroamphetamine)

___ Concerta (methylphenidate)

___ Contrave (bupropion/naltrexone)

___ Cotempla (methylphenidate)

___ Daytrana (methylphenidate)

___ Dexedrine (dextroamphetamine)

___ Evekeo (amphetamine Sulfate)

___ Focalin (dexmethylphenidate)

___ Focalin XR (dexmethylphenidate HCL)

___ Jornay PM (methylphenidate HCl)

___ Intuniv (guanfacine)

___ Metadate (methylp/hydrochloride)

Mood Stabilizers

___ Abilify (aripiprazole)

___ Chlorpromazine(thorazine)

___ Depakote/Depakene (valproic acid)

___ Fanapt (iloperidone)

___ Geodon (ziprasidone)

___ Haldol (haloperidol)

___ Invega (paliperidone)

___ Keppra (levetiracetam)

___ Lamictal (lamotrigine)

___ Latuda (lurasidone)

___ Lybalvi (olanzapine/ samidorphan)

___ Lithane, Lithobid (lithium)

___ Loxitane (loxapine)

Misc Sleep

____ Ambien (zolpidem)

____ Ambien CR (zolpidem CR)

____ Belsomra (suvorexant)

____ Clonidine (catapress)

____ Halcion (triazolam)

____ Intermezzo (zolpidem)

____ Lunesta (eszopiclone)

____ Melatonin

____ Restoril (temazepam)

____ Rozerem (ramelteon)

____ Silenor (doxepin)

____ Sonata (zaleplon)

____ Trazodone (oleptro)

____ Zolpimist (zolpidem)

Stimulants /Wake Promoting

____ Methylin (methylphenidate)

____ Mydayis (dextroamphetamine)

____ Quillichew (methylphenidate)

____ Quillivant XR (methylphenidate hydrochloride)

____ Ritalin (methylphenidate)

____ Saxenda (liraglutide)

____ Vyvanse (lisdexamfetamine)

____ Zenzedi (dextroamphetamine sulfate)

Antidepressants

____ Anafranil (clomipramine)

____ Celexa (citalopram)

____ Effexor (venlafaxine)

____ Fetzima (amitriptyline)

Mood Stabilizers

____ Navane (thiothixene)

____ Neurontin (gabapentin)

____ Rexulti (brexpiprazole)

____ Risperdal (risperidone)

____ Saphris (asenapine)

____ Seroquel XR (quetiapine)

____ Stavzor (valproic acid)

____ Symbyax (fluoxetine/ olanzapine)

____ Topamax (topiramate)

____ Trileptal (oxcarbazepine)

____ Zyprexa (olanzapine)

Anxiety Medications

_____ Ativan (lorazepam)

_____ Buspar (buspirone)

_____ Inderal (propranolol)

_____ Klonopin (clonazepam)

_____ Librium (chlordiazepoxide)

_____ Niravam (alprazolam)

_____ Valium (diazepam)

_____ Vistaril (hydroxyzine)

_____ Xanax (alprazolam)

Antidepressants

_____ Lexapro (escitalopram)

_____ Norpramin (desipramine)

_____ Pamelor (nortriptyline)

_____ Paxil (paroxetine)

_____ Pristiq (desvenlafaxine)

_____ Prozac (fluoxetine)

_____ Remeron (mirtazapine)

_____ Serzone (nefazodone)

_____ Sinequan (doxepin)

_____ Tofranil (imipramine)

_____ Trintellix (vortioxetine)

_____ Viibryd (vilazodone)

_____ Wellbutrin (bupropion)

_____ Zoloft (sertraline)

_____ Pexeva (paroxetine)

Appendix 4

Action Plan to "Wake Up to Narcolepsy"

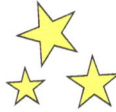

My Action Plan to "Wake Up to Narcolepsy"

Date _____

The top 10 things I learned from this book:

1

2)

3)

4)

5)

6)

7)

8)

9)

10)

The top 5 people I want to share this latest information with:

1)

2)

3)

4)

5)

<u>My top 5 action items:</u>

1)

2)

3)

4)

5)

About the Author

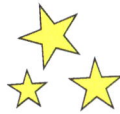

Dr. Debra Stultz is an author, professional speaker, and physician residing in Huntington, WV, where she is in private practice at Stultz Sleep & Behavioral Health. She graduated from Marshall University School of Medicine and completed her residency and fellowship with West Virginia University School of Medicine-Charleston Division.

Dr. Stultz has been a long-time advocate in the treatment of Narcolepsy, with many presentations and research papers over the years to advance the awareness of this disorder. She has recorded video lectures on Narcolepsy with the *Psychiatric Times* and *Neurology Live*. She has done a live nationwide broadcast from HBO studios in New York City entitled "Navigating Narcolepsy: A Case-Based Clinical Series." She has written a chapter in the *American Academy of Sleep Medicine Case Book of Sleep Medicine* entitled "Navigating Narcolepsy During Pregnancy." She is a nationwide speaker on the topics of Narcolepsy, insomnia, and the use of Transcranial Magnetic Stimulation (TMS) for resistant depression. Dr. Stultz is board-certified in Psychiatry, a distinguished Fellow of the Clinical TMS Society, certified in Behavioral Sleep Medicine, and a Diplomate of the American Board of Sleep Medicine. She is also the editor of the CTMSS "TMS Today" newsletter. Dr. Stultz and two of her writing partners, Laura B. Herpel MD and Lewis J. Kass MD, have created a "Narcolepsy Assessment & Progress Screener" to aid in the evaluation and progress during the treatment of this disorder, with the addition recently of a pediatric version.

Her video presentations with the *Psychiatric Times Case-Based Psych Perspectives Broadcasts* are entitled "Expert Perspectives on the Management of Narcolepsy and its Comorbidities" and "Narcolepsy Management and the Roles Neurologists and Psychiatrist Play." The *NeurologyLive* videos are entitled "Unmet Needs in Narcolepsy and Clinical Pearls." Research poster presentations at the American Academy of Sleep Medicine on Narcolepsy over the years include: "A one-year observational early access pitolisant study of excessive daytime sleepiness in Narcolepsy," "Narcolepsy associated with a history of a head injury: A retrospective review," "Post-traumatic Narcolepsy in 9 military veterans with a history of a head injury," and a 2022 late-breaking abstract accepted entitled "Increased female prevalence of depression in patients with Narcolepsy and co-existing depression: a 10-year review." She also had a research publication entitled "Assessment of Clinical Response to Narcolepsy Treatment: Challenges and Best Practices" in *The Research Post*.

Dr. Stultz is a single Mother of two children whom she adores and one wonderful son-in-law. She is a devoted daughter, sister, friend, and physician. She has an extended circle of friends she calls family. She is surrounded by a talented, enthusiastic, and supportive office staff. She enjoys writing and photography.

Dr. Stultz is passionate about educating others about sleep and psychiatric disorders, especially treatment-resistant depression, Transcranial Magnetic Stimulation (TMS), sports psychiatry, head injuries, insomnia, and Narcolepsy. Dr. Stultz can be reached at (304)-733-5380. For more information, visit Stultz Sleep & Behavioral Health at www.drdebrastultz.com

Offers

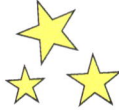

Offer #1

Windshield/School/Work Placard

I have repeatedly stated that "Napping is Necessary" in treating Narcolepsy. We have created a placard to place around you while napping at school/work or to put on your dashboard if you are napping in your car before driving or when you have pulled off beside the road to sleep. I feel this will help alert others why you are there and prevent alarm. It will also help to avoid disruptions to your nap.

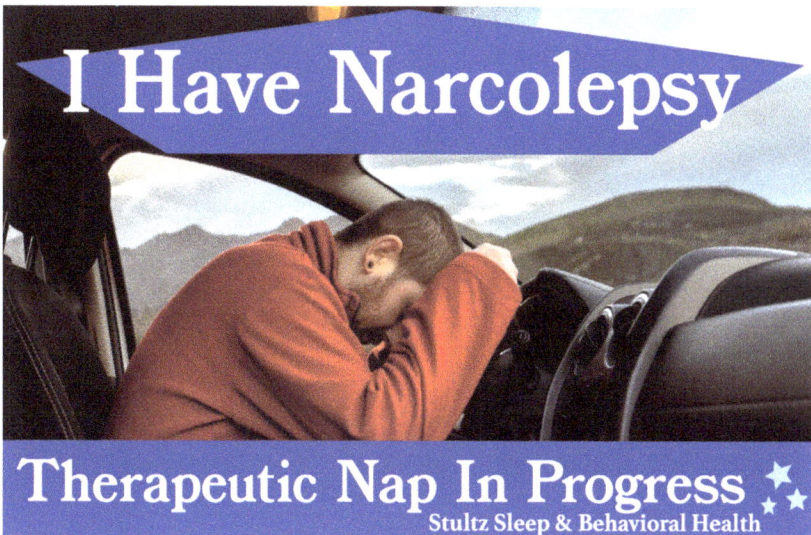

School Nap Placard

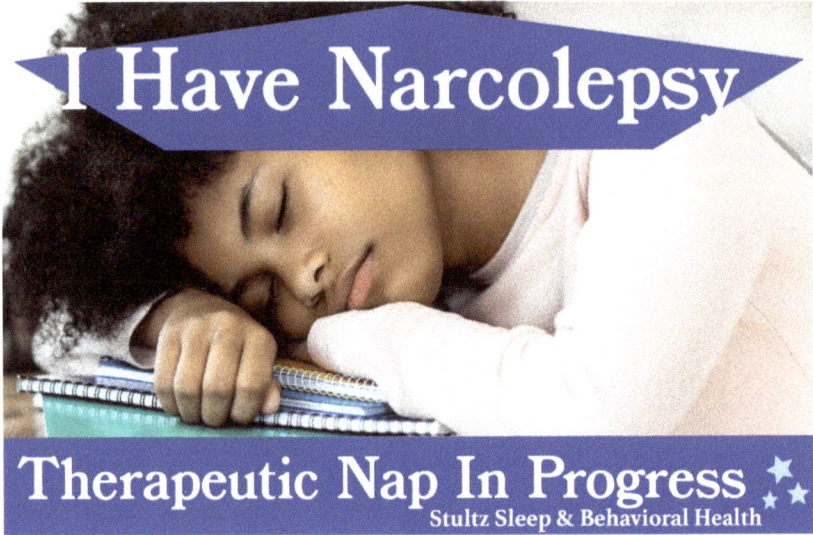

Ordering information:

This can be ordered at my website: www.drdebrastultz.com under "Products."

Offer #2

Narcolepsy Badge

We suggest you wear a medical alert bracelet or a badge identifying yourself as having Narcolepsy and informing others of what to do. The internet has various med alert bracelets you can order. Below is one possible example that you can order from our office explaining both the sleepiness and cataplexy presentations of Narcolepsy to others.

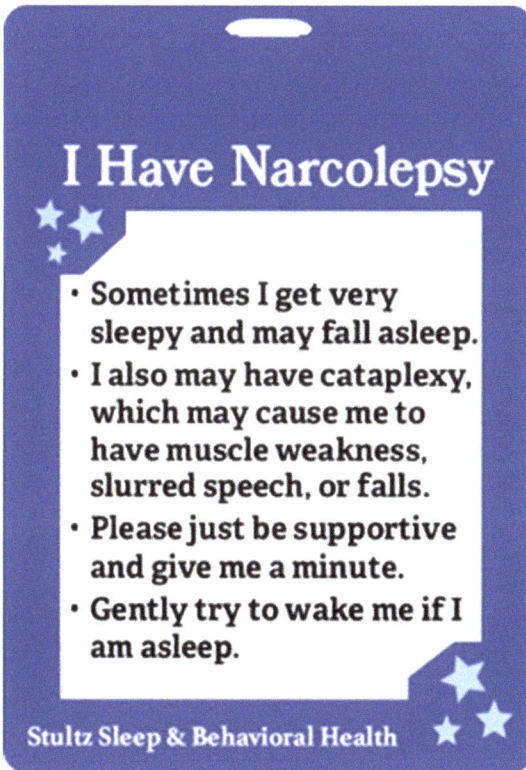

Ordering information:

This, too, can be ordered at my website: www.dr.debrastultz.com under "Products."

DR. DEBRA STULTZ

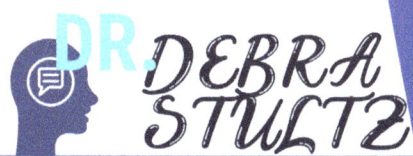

SPEAKER PRESENTATIONS

Dr. Stultz is an enthusiastic, sincere, inspiring, and motivating speaker to providers, patients, students, sleep fellows, residents, and therapists. She shares her 30+ years of experience as a Psychiatrist, Author, Internationally-known Speaker, and Sleep Physician.

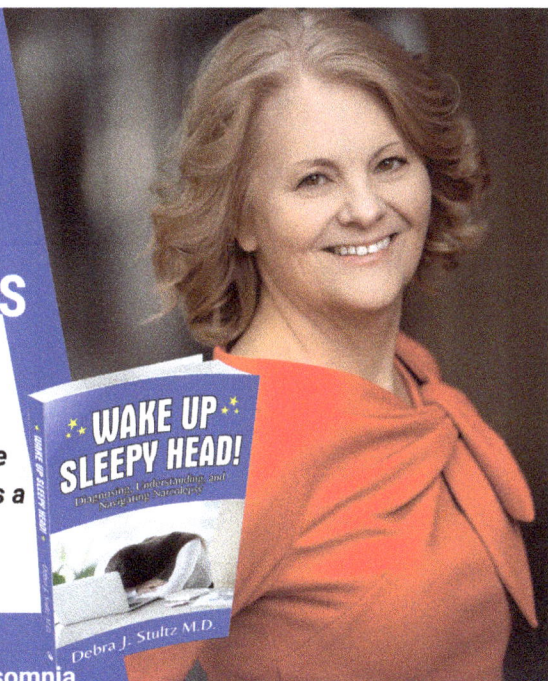

WAKE UP SLEEPY HEAD!
Diagnosing, Understanding and Navigating Narcolepsy

Debra J. Stultz M.D.

✓ **Narcolepsy & Idiopathic Hypersomnia**
- Treatment and Diagnosis of Narcolepsy and other Causes of Hypersomnia
- Pharmacological Options, Behavioral Treatments and Family Interventions
- Pediatric, Adolescent, Adult, and Elderly Presentations of Narcolepsy

✓ **Treatment-Resistant Depression**
- Identifying All of the Pieces of the Puzzle Contributing to Resistant Depression
- New and Novel Treatments of Depression

✓ **Transcranial Magnetic Stimulation**
- Non-Medication Treatment for Depression, Migraines, and OCD
- Upcoming Indications for TMS Use in Substance Abuse, Pain, Strokes, etc.

✓ **Diagnosing Sleep Disorders**
- Comprehensive Evaluation and Diagnosis Contributing to Insomnia and Hypersomnia
- Pharmacologic and Behavioral Treatments of Insomnia and Other Sleep Disorders

Lectures can be provided in-person or online for events, such as conferences, promotional gatherings, seminars, and private events.

📞 (304) 733-5380
🌐 www.drdebrastultz.com
📍 6171 Childers Rd., Barboursville, WV 25504
✉ wvsleepdoc@outlook.com

Stultz Sleep
& Behavioral Health

Notes

www.ingramcontent.com/pod-product-compliance
Lightning Source LLC
Chambersburg PA
CBHW052111030426
42335CB00025B/2938